Nursing in the Storm

Denise Danna, DNS, RN, is Associate Dean for Professional Services, Community Activities, and Advanced Nursing Practice Education, Louisiana State University Health Sciences Center, School of Nursing, New Orleans. For 32 years, Dr. Danna worked at Memorial Medical Center, New Orleans, holding several leadership positions, including Chief Nursing Officer for 15 years. She is an active member of the American Nurses Association, American Organization of Nurse Executives, National League for Nursing, and Sigma Theta Tau International. She is a fellow in the American College of Health Care Executives. She has recently authored a book chapter on management and leadership issues, published several articles on disaster preparedness, and is a reviewer for Nursing Outlook. Dr. Danna is currently the President of the Louisiana Nurses Association.

Sandra E. Cordray, MA, MJ, holds a Master of Arts from the University of Wales where she studied from 1986–1987 at the university's Centre for Journalism Studies. She also received a Master of Journalism from Louisiana State University in 1989. For three decades she has worked in the fields of marketing and media relations for health care and educational organizations, holding management positions at the hospital and regional levels in New Orleans, Texas, and south Florida. During her nine years at Memorial Medical Center in New Orleans she handled marketing and media relations and served as public information officer for the hurricane season. She serves on the board of directors for New Orleans Artists Against Hunger and Homelessness. A native of Biloxi, Mississippi, she was raised on the Mississippi Gulf Coast where her sisters and brothers still reside. Hurricane Camille was the first major hurricane she experienced.

The authors will donate a portion of the proceeds from this book to support nursing education programs for disaster preparedness.

Nursing in the Storm

Voices from Hurricane Katrina

DENISE DANNA, DNS, RN
SANDRA E. CORDRAY, MA, MJ

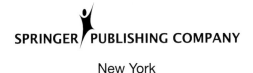

SPRINGER PUBLISHING COMPANY

New York

Springer Publishing Company, LLC   *Acquisitions Editor: Allan Graubard*
11 West 42nd Street   *Project Manager: Mark Frazier*
New York, NY 10036   *Cover Design: Mimi Flow*
www.springerpub.com   *Composition: Apex*

10 11 12 / 5 4 3   E-book ISBN: 978-0-8261-1838-7

The authors and the publisher of this Work have made every effort to use sources believed to be reliable to provide information that is accurate and compatible with the standards generally accepted at the time of publication. Because medical science is continually advancing, our knowledge base continues to expand. Therefore, as new information becomes available, changes in procedures become necessary. We recommend that the reader always consult current research and specific institutional policies before performing any clinical procedure. The authors and publisher shall not be liable for any special, consequential, or exemplary damages resulting, in whole or in part, from the readers' use of, or reliance on, the information contained in this book. The publisher has no responsibility for the persistence or accuracy of URLs for external or third-party Internet Web sites referred to in this publication and does not guarantee that any content on such Web sites is, or will remain, accurate or appropriate.

Library of Congress Cataloging-in-Publication Data

Danna, Denise.
   Nursing in the storm : voices from Hurricane Katrina / Denise Danna, Sandra E. Cordray.
        p. ; cm.
   Includes bibliographical references and index.
   ISBN 978-0-8261-1837-0 (alk. paper)
   1. Disaster nursing—Louisiana—New Orleans.   2. Nurses—Louisiana—New Orleans.   3. Hurricane Katrina, 2005.   I. Cordray, Sandra E.   II. Title.
   [DNLM: 1. Cyclones—New Orleans—Personal Narratives.   2. Nurses—New Orleans—Personal Narratives.   3. Disasters—New Orleans—Personal Narratives.   4. Hospitals—New Orleans—Personal Narratives.   5. Nurse's Role—New Orleans—Personal Narratives.   6. Nursing Care—New Orleans—Personal Narratives.   WZ 112.5.N8 D188n 2009]
   RT108.D36 2009
   610.73'490976335—dc22   2009040881

Printed in the United States of America by Hamilton Printing.

Cover photos: (top right) by Scarlett Welch-Nakajima; (radar image) courtesy of University of Wisconsin Cooperative Institute for Meterological Satellite Studies.
The photo on page vii is an aerial photo taken from a U.S. Navy helicopter that shows the flooded downtown area of New Orleans following Hurricane Katrina. In the center of the photograph is the Louisiana Superdome, its roof peeled back from hurricane-force winds. Photo by U.S. Navy.

To the nurses who served on the front lines during and following Hurricane Katrina and to all who were touched by this storm. You were not alone.

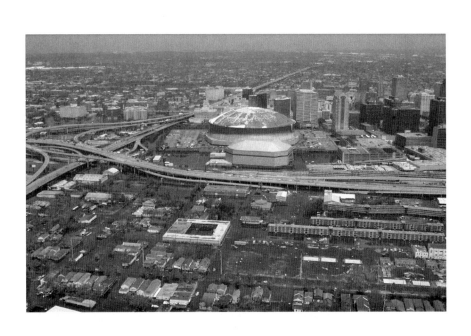

Contents

Foreword

This is a compelling, first-person story as told by Katrina nurses. The second chapter, which describes Charity Hospital, demonstrates their courage, commitment, and American spirit. These nurses adapted to, and overcame, near-wartime conditions with the courage of Clara Barton and the grace of Mother Theresa. I think the ultimate human experience is to be able to save someone's life. These nurses are to be commended for all the lives they saved. Charity Hospital saved my life as a young boy. I am sorry we did not get to help you sooner.
—Lieutenant General Russel Honoré

Following the devastation of Hurricane Katrina in summer 2005, Lieutenant General Russel L. Honoré, U.S. Army (retired), was commander of Joint Task Force–Katrina, which was responsible for coordinating military relief efforts across the Gulf Coast. His experience planning response operations in the wake of disasters is extensive and includes efforts in response to hurricanes Floyd in 1999; Lili and Isadore in 2002; Isabel in 2003; and Charley, Frances, Ivan, and Jeanne in 2004.

After more than 37 years of distinguished service, he retired from the army in January 2008 and embarked on a new mission: creating a *culture of preparedness* in America. He is author of *Survival: How a Culture of Preparedness Can Save You and Your Family From Disasters.* The book is both a personal memoir and account of the events of Hurricane Katrina and a guide on disaster preparedness. General Honoré is CNN's lead expert on disaster preparedness and is a senior scientist with the Gallup Organization. He is a visiting professor at the Emory University School of Public Health and an assistant clinical professor at Vanderbilt School of Nursing.

Preface

The tragedy of Hurricane Katrina drew all eyes to the New Orleans area and dominated the international media for weeks. The hurricane necessitated a national response that federal, state, and local officials were unprepared to provide, but the nurses working at six hospitals—Charity Hospital and University Hospital of the Medical Center of Louisiana at New Orleans, Lindy Boggs Medical Center, Memorial Medical Center, Pendleton Memorial Methodist Hospital, and Chalmette Medical Center—had a unique view of the tragedy. In all the books, thousands of news stories, and hours of television coverage, their story has not been told—until now.

On Monday, August 29, 2005, at 6:10 A.M. Central Daylight Time, Hurricane Katrina made landfall (its second) as a strong Category 3 storm in southeastern Louisiana, near Buras. The eye of the hurricane passed slightly to the east of New Orleans and brought with it strong winds and vast storm surges. The city's levee system had over 50 failures, which led to floodwaters drowning almost 80% of New Orleans and transforming hospitals into islands, where resources and communications gradually deteriorated (American Society of Civil Engineers, 2007).

At the front lines were nurses, who were subsequently thrust into third world conditions. Maintaining patient care with no electricity to run life-saving medical devices, air-conditioners, elevators, lights, and pumps during this period brought special challenges, particularly for critical patients and those patients confined to bed. With systems down, records and physician orders had to be maintained manually. Food had to be rationed. So did supplies and other essential services needed by patients. After the storm, the hospitals also became refuges for numerous residents who were displaced by the flooding.

In the months immediately following Hurricane Katrina, the idea for this book was sown, as the authors tried to process what they had experienced at one of the hospitals incapacitated by the disaster and comprehend the ramifications of the hurricane's impact on the nursing profession in the greater New Orleans area.

The nurses' profiles in this book are based on information obtained from direct interviews conducted in person or by telephone. Any statement in quotations was recorded in a formal interview and represents that individual's recollection of events between August 29, 2005 and September 3, 2005. Additional interviews were conducted with Sandy Rosenthal, the founder and director of Levees.org, and with an administrative designated regional coordinator for hospital emergency preparedness and response in Louisiana Region 1, the greater New Orleans area. The quoted statements are the opinions and recollections of the people who expressed them.

For every nurse at these hospitals, there is a story. The connective tissue that binds them is the fact that they were on the front lines during a catastrophic event. The infrastructure needed to provide care to their patients no longer existed—and, for many of them, neither did their homes. Some have kept their experiences locked silently away—what they witnessed is too painful to put into words and would take too much effort; others have shared their experiences privately with colleagues and family; and some nurses have been able to translate their experiences with Hurricane Katrina into discussion at national and international nursing conferences around the world.

We are indebted to these nurses for sharing their personal accounts of a catastrophic experience. They are among thousands of nurses who endured conditions that left a devastating imprint. Hurricane Katrina became a defining moment in the development of the way they and others perceive nursing and emergency response during a major disaster.

We salute the courage of these nurses. They have given voice to what they witnessed at the water's edge so that others will know that they were not alone.

At Springer Publishing, our thanks go to Allan Graubard, senior acquisitions editor, for suggesting the book to us and for advising us along the way, and to Brian O'Connor, assistant editor.

Thanks also go to Elizabeth Rosen, PhD; Linda Easterlin, for her helpful suggestions; Carl Baribault, for his words of encouragement; and our families, for their unwavering faith and support.

It is our hope that the collective voices in this book will continue the dialogue, helping us to understand the way things were pre-Katrina and giving us the courage to change them for the better in the future.

A very brief history of nursing in New Orleans precedes the heart of the book.

Hope has two beautiful daughters. Their names are anger and courage: anger that things are the way they are; courage to make them the way they ought to be.

—St. Augustine

1 History of Nursing in New Orleans

The foundations of nursing in New Orleans are steeped in a long, rich history associated with missionaries and several religious orders of sisters. Nursing by the religious extends back to the 1700s, when nine Ursuline sisters arrived in New Orleans from France, initially to care for the sick, then for children, and to establish orphanages. The Sisters of Ursula established the first convent in New Orleans in 1752. The Sisters of Mercy, who arrived in New Orleans from St. Louis, Missouri, in 1869, also visited the sick in their homes and provided an educational foundation for children and adults.

Known for their skill in providing nursing care to people in the public hospitals in France, the Daughters of Charity also came to New Orleans over 250 years ago to care for the sick and poor at Charity Hospital. In fact, the Daughters of Charity were instrumental in providing and creating health care services in New Orleans. In 1859, they built their own hospital, which became known as Hotel Dieu (House of God). Then, in 1861, the Daughters of Charity opened a facility for patients afflicted with mental illness and named it DePaul Hospital—this hospital is still used for psychiatric services today (Salvaggio, 1992).

NURSING EDUCATION

During the late 1800s, as medical schools were being opened in New Orleans, it became obvious to hospital administrators that nursing schools were a possible source of cheap labor with which to staff hospitals. Thus the vice president of Charity Hospital's board of directors, Dr. Daniel Holliday, proposed the creation of a formalized nursing school at Charity Hospital. Dr. Holliday had obtained enough funding for the nursing school, but the hospital's board of directors wanted the Daughters of Charity's approval to move forward. Unfortunately, the sisters refused because they had not been included in the planning. As Sister Agnes, mother superior, stated,

> In the nature of things, having in view the object proposed by the establishment of the training school, the Sister Superior [should] not exercise the same absolute authority over the matron and the pupils, which is now exercised over all other persons connected with the hospital, except its officers; and the oneness of authority is in our opinion essential to proper discipline, as well as to prevent grave abuses and evils which but little reflection will suggest. (Salvaggio, 1992, p. 89)

Ten years later, due to continued pressure and complaints that medical services were not improving at Charity Hospital, the board of directors developed a set of bylaws for establishing a school of nursing. A layperson was selected as the nursing school's first director: Mary Agnes O'Donnell, who was a Bellevue Nursing School graduate. It is important to note that authority over and control of issues relating to discipline were still in the hands of the mother superior. In 1897, seven sisters graduated in the first class of the Charity School of Nursing (Salvaggio, 1992).

Over the early years, nursing students served as the major source of manpower for the hospital. Although the pay was minimal, the education and training the students received was excellent, and the Charity School of Nursing graduate was often recruited and sought after by other hospitals—a situation that prevails even today. Since the inception of the Charity School of Nursing, several sisters have served as director, including Sister Stanislaus and Sister Henrietta Guyot. These leaders laid the foundation for the successes realized, and advancements made, in nursing education and the profession of nursing in New Orleans.

Sister Stanislaus's accomplishments include the development of the curriculum for the first bachelor of science degree in nursing education provided at the Louisiana State University (LSU) Extension Division in Baton Rouge. In 1916, Sister Stanislaus also started the School of Anesthesia at Charity Hospital. For over 60 years, from 1883 to 1946, she served the sick and poor of New Orleans (Dawes & Nolan, 2004).

Sister Henrietta Guyot was associated with nursing education for over 28 years in New Orleans, specifically with the Charity School of Nursing. She began her career at Charity Hospital and the Charity School of Nursing in 1927, graduating from Charity's 3-year diploma program in 1930 (Dawes & Nolan, 2004). While serving as an assistant instructor in the nursing school, she began attending college classes at LSU Extension Division, Baton Rouge. She received a bachelor of science degree in nursing education in 1933 and obtained her master's degree in nursing from Catholic University 2 years later (Dawes & Nolan, 2004). In 1937, the nursing program was transferred to the LSU School of Medicine, which was under the control of physicians and where Sister Guyot was a full professor (Dawes & Nolan, 2004).

Sister Guyot was responsible for the expansion and improvement of the curriculum of the Nurse Anesthesia Program, in response to higher accreditation and educational standards. She was involved with the construction of a new 400-bed nursing school in 1940, which was located adjacent to a new 2,500-plus-bed Charity Hospital, making Charity one of the largest hospitals in the country (Dawes & Nolan, 2004). Sister Guyot developed a nursing services policy book that provided guidelines and standardization for nurses to use in their practice.

During Sister Guyot's leadership, the school of nursing was reorganized; she was one of the first to identify the need to separate the then dual role of director of nursing service and the school of nursing into two positions, ensuring the education of future nurses for service and providing quality care to patients by educated and trained practitioners (Dawes & Nolan, 2004).

Certainly not averse to controversy, Sister Guyot was involved in the following innovations: She encouraged fathers of newborns to attend the delivery; integrated the New Orleans District Nurses Association; promoted the push for higher education for nurses; and was responsible for securing traineeship funds for nurses in cardiovascular disorders (Dawes & Nolan, 2004).

The Louisiana Department of Nursing, in 1955, reported that they planned to disband the standard nursing curriculum and establish a 4-year baccalaureate degree in nursing beginning in 1958, with future plans to develop a master's program in nursing curriculum. In the early 1980s, the Charity School of Nursing diploma school was closed and transitioned into an associate degree program under the auspices of Delgado Community College. There is little question that Sister Guyot influenced the character of education, the profession of nursing, and the public health of the people of the state of Louisiana (Dawes & Nolan, 2004).

NURSING REGULATION

In 1904, licensure for nurses took a first step through the creation of a nursing organization, the Louisiana State Nurses Association (LSNA), in New Orleans. Sixty-five nurses were interested; 33 nurses actually came to the first meeting, and 32 more nurses sent letters of endorsement (Hanggi-Myers, 1996). The LSNA and its members proposed the first bill for licensure, modeled after the State of Maryland Licensure Act, in 1904. The bill was unsuccessful because its five-member board consisted only of women, and women were not allowed to hold public office or vote (Hanggi-Myers, 1996).

The nurses of the LSNA continued to educate health care professionals and the public on the development of regulations for nurses. Over the next 8 years, women still did not gain the right to hold public office or vote, so the LSNA had no other choice but to accept governance from the physician-run State Board of Examiners (Hanggi-Myers, 1996). Nonetheless, Act 138, whereby the Louisiana State Board of Nursing came into existence, was adopted by the legislature and signed by Governor Hall on July 10, 1912 (Hanggi-Myers, 1996).

In 1922, Act 138 was amended by Act 46, which stipulated that the Board of Nursing should consist of two nurse members and three physician members, and by Act 4, passed in 1926, which increased the number of nurse members on the board from two to three (Hanggi-Myers, 1996).

In 1942, the regulations were amended by Act 93, which officially changed the name of the Board of Nursing to the Louisiana State Board of Nurse Examiners. Registered nurses were slowly taking control over nursing practice. Today, the Nurse Practice Act is incorporated into the Revised Statutes under Title 37, Chapter 11, Part I, Registered Nurses.

2

Medical Center of Louisiana at New Orleans: Charity and University Hospitals

Two hundred seventy-six years ago, in March 1736, a French seaman and boatbuilder named Jean Louis donated funds to open L'Hospital des Pauvres de la Charité (Hospital of the Poor). Horrified that the poor were being turned away from the Royal Hospital (whose only poor patients were those who had served in the military), Jean Louis determined to make some provisions for care of the indigent population. So, on May 10, 1736, a house at Chartres and Bienville streets became the first Charity Hospital. The hospital quickly outgrew its space, and in 1743, at the edge of the city, in an area known today as Basin Street, the second Charity Hospital was constructed (Salvaggio, 1992).

Charity has a history with hurricanes. A third Charity Hospital had to be built in 1785 after two hurricanes decimated it: one in 1778, which significantly damaged the hospital, and the other in 1779, which totally destroyed the hospital. The third hospital was built only after many years of the city's poor suffering without care and services. This third hospital was named Hospital of St. Charles (San Carlo Hospital), in honor of King Charles III of Spain. One of New Orleans's streets, Almonaster, was named after the man responsible for building the third hospital (Salvaggio, 1992). In 1809, another unfortunate event—this time a catastrophic fire—destroyed the third Charity Hospital.

The fourth hospital, built during the following 5 years after that fire, was relocated to Canal Street, then actually swampland that sat next to the cemeteries. This hospital was considered a very large facility then, providing care for 120 patients, but after several years, it was found to have deplorable conditions (Salvaggio, 1992).

Due to the enormous increase in the city's population, a fifth Charity Hospital was built in 1833. This fifth hospital—because of its size, physical structure, and number of beds—was considered a city landmark (Salvaggio, 1992). The sixth and current Charity Hospital was built in 1939 at its present site on Tulane Avenue after a personal visit from President Theodore Roosevelt. The new Charity Hospital opened with 2,650 beds, along with a 14-floor school of nursing. It was the second oldest hospital in the country at the time, and the oldest continuously operating hospital bearing the same name in the United States (Salvaggio, 1992).

Caring for the indigent, whether native born or European immigrants, and responding to the needs of the public has been the mission of Charity Hospital since its founding. Over the years, Charity Hospital had faced lingering financial pressures, political favoritism, problems with poor staffing, overcrowding, an unsanitary environment, and poor or nonexistent equipment and supplies. Being governed by many authorities, including the Daughters of Charity and the state, also placed pressures on the hospital, compromising its work for the community that it served.

University Hospital was opened as Hotel Dieu Hospital in 1859, over 100 years after Charity Hospital. It was founded, owned, and operated by the Daughters of Charity, an American order of nuns affiliated with Elizabeth Ann Bayley Seton of France. The name Hotel Dieu means "House of God" in French. Hotel Dieu kept its doors open and operational during the Civil War and through two yellow fever epidemics (University Hospital, 1996–2007).

A new Hotel Dieu Hospital was built in 1924 and, in 1972, was replaced with another new building, still located on Perdido Street in New Orleans. In 1992, Louisiana governor Edwin Edwards requested that the Daughters of Charity sell Hotel Dieu to the state. At that time, Hotel Dieu Hospital was renamed University Hospital (University Hospital, 1996–2007).

The Medical Center of Louisiana at New Orleans (MCLNO; both Charity and University hospitals) suffered major destruction due to Hurricane Katrina in August 2005. Both campuses were closed after Katrina, which resulted in a major loss in health care services for the underserved and underinsured in the city. In addition, the only Level 1 Trauma Center in the city at the time was closed.

With a tremendous need for health care services in the New Orleans area after Hurricane Katrina, the MCLNO, along with its trauma care center, was relocated to the U.S. Naval ship USNS *Comfort*, which was docked at New Orleans on the Mississippi River. It had been brought to New Orleans on September 29, 2005, after Hurricane Katrina, to serve as a temporary hospital. Physicians and nurses from Charity Hospital were oriented and participated in the care of the sick on the ship until its departure.

Aptly named "The Spirit of Charity," emergency services were also established in military tents in a parking lot beside the damaged University Hospital on October 10, 2005. Just over a month later, the emergency services, tents and all, were relocated to the massive Ernest N. Morial Convention Center, the hall where so many people had waited for evacuation following the flooding of New Orleans. Emergency services personnel remained at the Convention Center, often seeing over 1,000 patients per day, until the services were moved again to a nearby vacant Lord and Taylor department store several blocks away from the MCLNO. Physicians and nurses continued to see large numbers of patients. Patients who needed hospitalization were transferred to one of the local hospitals that had not experienced flooding or to another Louisiana State University (LSU) system hospital outside New Orleans.

Trauma services for Charity Hospital were established on April 24, 2006, at Elmwood Medical Center in nearby Jefferson Parish. On November 17, 2006, Interim LSU Public Hospital reopened at the Perdido Street location with 75 inpatient beds and basic emergency services. As the remodeled trauma services and additional trauma ICU [intensive care unit] beds were completed, the trauma program returned to Interim LSU Public Hospital on February 22, 2007, and was reaccredited in December 2008. Ambulatory services opened in October 2005. Currently various clinics are operated from the vacated Lord and Taylor department store and other buildings in the health care system complex. Today, Interim LSU Public Hospital is operational at 224 inpatient beds, and Charity Hospital—the "Big Free"—still hovers over the city, closed but not forgotten by many.

At the January 23, 2009, hearing by the House Appropriations Committee, discussion continued on the future of Charity Hospital. The state plans call for building a $1.2 billion academic medical complex in lower Mid-City. The plans include the expenditure of $54 million to buy homes and businesses within a 70-acre footprint bordered by Canal

Street, South Rocheblave Street, Tulane Avenue, and South Claiborne Avenue. It has been met with resistance from neighborhood residents who are rebuilding their flooded homes with Road Home grants that are financed by taxpayer dollars. The Foundation for Historical Louisiana has offered an alternative plan for gutting the shuttered Charity Hospital and turning it into a teaching hospital.

On August 28, 2009, one day before the 4-year anniversary of Hurricane Katriana, Louisiana governor Bobby Jindal and leaders from LSU System and Tulane University signed a memorandum of understanding. The agreement signals steps forward to build a new teaching hospital to replace the former Charity Hospital.

When the levees breached on August 29, 2005, approximately 1,000 employees and patients were stranded in the Charity and University hospitals, with floodwaters 8–10 feet deep surrounding the buildings. The last patients and staff were finally evacuated on September 3, 2005, and dispersed to locations ranging from Atlanta to San Antonio.

Seven nurses recount what they experienced during their last days at Charity and University hospitals before the closure of Charity, one of the country's oldest continuously operating hospitals.

Olander Holloway

I am still amazed at the selfless dedication of the staff. It was 6 days of hell. It was unbelievable. For 6 days staff cared for patients on their knees.

Olander Holloway, RN, graduated from the Orleans Parish Practical Nursing Program in January 1968. She worked in the labor and delivery unit at Charity Hospital as a licensed practical nurse for 3 years before going back to school. She attended Charity School of Nursing and graduated in 1974. Her nursing experience as a registered nurse included labor and delivery, medical/surgical, intensive care, ambulatory care, clinics, and emergency, all at Charity Hospital. She returned to school and received a bachelor's of science degree in nursing (BSN) from Loyola University, New Orleans, in 1983. In 1985, she attended Loyola Law School and graduated in 1989 with a JD degree. She was the director of emergency services from 1985 until she retired in December 2005, after Hurricane Katrina.

When Olander reports to work at Charity Hospital before seven o'clock on Sunday morning, August 28, 2005, the routine for emergency preparedness was one that had become second nature to her during a 35-year nursing career. She had worked for every tropical storm, every hurricane. As a member of the hospital's activation team, she is one of two nursing administrators reporting to work. At Charity Hospital and the nearby sister facility, University Hospital, there is an equal level of staffing for the emergency room, with two head nurses and a supervisor at each campus.

Establishing an Incident Command Center is a scenario that unfolds at all hospitals in the path of the hurricane and one with which hospital staff members are familiar from their participation in hospital emergency preparedness drills. The Incident Command System was developed in the 1970s by an interagency task force working in cooperation with local, state, and federal agencies called Firefighting Resources of California Organized for Potential Emergencies (Firescape), organized to combat wildfires. In February 2003, the Homeland Security Presidential Directive 5 was issued by President George W. Bush to create the National Incident Management System (Federal Emergency Management Agency [FEMA], 2008).

The Incident Command System organizational chart includes the positions of incident commander, public information officer, safety officer, liaisons officer, medical/technical specialist, and other positions for finance, logistics, operations, and planning (FEMA, 2008). Olander has always been on Team A, the first tier of employees who worked during hurricanes. When her children were younger, during some storms, she brought them with her to the hospital, where they stayed in the day care area. For less severe storms, they stayed at home with her husband, Robert, who would never go to the hospital with her. But this storm was different.

"I remember that something just didn't feel right. I don't know what it was, but I told him, 'You need to come with me to the hospital. They're talking about it being bad. You need to come.' But he was going to stay at home—him and the guy next door. My neighbor was a nurse also. Her husband and my husband wanted to stay home, but when my husband went out and saw the guy next door packing up, he asked, 'Where are you going?' and my neighbor said, 'Well, I was going to stay, but Felicia was upset and she wants to take the kids out of here. She has two little ones. We are going to go.' So my husband looked around and the rest of our neighbors were gone. He said, 'If my neighbor is going, I have to get out of here.' He made it back to the hospital by five."

By that time all staff have their assignments. Olander and her colleagues anticipate being at the hospital for a few days after the storm.

"When I first got there, I wanted to get everyone settled down and make schedules. Normally we'd work 12-hour shifts in the emergency room."

"Medical Center of Louisiana at New Orleans' disaster plan was that all emergency services located at University Hospital would shut down, but I wanted the supervisors and the head nurses to assign two people to each department so we had coverage for the two campuses. We divided the staff into 6-hour shifts. Initially, medical services were supposed to shut down at University Hospital and relocate at Charity Hospital, since it was a much larger hospital. But of course things changed, and that did not happen. We needed to make sure that we had the same level of staff on both campuses. After that, most of that day was getting supplies in, making sure everything was in place."

The anticipation among the staff is that this storm would be a routine matter with the temporary loss of electricity, where the main elevators would not be operational, but then a resumption of hospital functions was expected. The relief Team B (the staff who come in after the storm to relieve the current employees who had worked during the hurricane) would report and assume the assignments from Olander and her colleagues.

Sleeping quarters for the nursing staff are located at the walk-in clinic, an area used for minor emergencies. Olander and her husband sleep in her office. Nursing staff, family members, and patients number over 900. The patient population is more than 400. There are 50 critically ill patients at University Hospital. The emergency room—the trauma and medical emergency rooms—has nearly 70 patients on the day of the storm. On Sunday, August 28, the hospital determines a cutoff time for discharging patients to decrease the patient population as part of the hospital's emergency preparedness plan.

"I always felt bad about that," Olander shares. "We kept looking at decreasing the patient population, but the patients that we had, where were they going to go? I mean we were getting to the point you just as well as let all the patients stay here."

One challenge the staff has is trying to reach families who had left the city to ask them to return to get their family members who are patients. "Most of those [patients] needed to be here. They needed some type of care. We did have a few homeless patients who had no other place to go, so they came to the hospital for shelter."

By Sunday, Hurricane Katrina is a Category 5 storm and 12 hours away from landfall. That evening, the emergency room (ER) staff receive two major trauma cases. One is a young man with multiple gunshot wounds. Olander thinks it was odd that while everyone was worrying about the storm, "here they are shooting each other. What bar is open when there is a storm? We also had a stabbing victim. The gunshot patient had been shot a number of times. When he went to surgery we still had elevator service. The stabbing victim was a domestic issue. We also had an elderly lady who came in the middle of the night—a heart attack. She was one of the patients who expired. During that time, I think the emergency room only lost three patients, and she was one; but her death was not related to the conditions in the hospital. There were a couple of patients in [intensive care] that had expired."

Meanwhile, reports of Hurricane Katrina become more ominous:

KATRINA IS MOVING TOWARD THE NORTH NEAR 15 MPH . . . AND THIS MOTION IS FORECAST TO CONTINUE TODAY. A GRADUAL TURN TOWARD THE NORTH-NORTHEAST AT A SLIGHTLY FASTER FORWARD SPEED IS EXPECTED LATER TONIGHT AND ON TUESDAY. ON THE FORECAST TRACK . . . KATRINA WILL MOVE ONSHORE THE SOUTHEASTERN LOUISIANA COAST JUST EAST OF GRAND ISLE THIS MORNING . . . AND REACH THE LOUISIANA-MISSISSIPPI BORDER AREA THIS AFTERNOON. CONDITIONS WILL CONTINUE TO STEADILY DETERIORATE OVER CENTRAL AND SOUTHEASTERN LOUISIANA . . . SOUTHERN MISSISSIPPI . . . AND SOUTHERN ALABAMA THROUGHOUT THE DAY. MAXIMUM SUSTAINED WINDS ARE NEAR 150 MPH . . . 240 M/HR . . . WITH HIGHER GUSTS. KATRINA IS A STRONG CATEGORY FOUR HURRICANE ON THE SAFFIR-SIMPSON SCALE. SOME FLUCTUATIONS IN STRENGTH ARE LIKELY PRIOR TO LANDFALL . . . BUT KATRINA IS EXPECTED TO MAKE LANDFALL AS A CATEGORY FOUR HURRICANE. WINDS AFFECTING THE UPPER FLOORS OF HIGH-RISE BUILDINGS WILL BE SIGNIFICANTLY STRONGER THAN THOSE NEAR GROUND LEVEL. (National Hurricane Center, 2005a)

On Monday, August 29, at 6:10 A.M., Hurricane Katrina makes landfall near Buras, Louisiana. By then, the hurricane has weakened to a Category 3 storm. Its highest winds are 112 mph. Forty miles to the north of Buras, the winds are 60 mph, and the first flooding of the greater New Orleans area has begun. Lake Borgne, east of New Orleans, has a storm surge that peaked around 7:00 A.M. Forty-five minutes later, two sections of the levee along the eastern side of the southern end of the Industrial Canal collapse. The lower Ninth Ward is flooding.

That morning, when Olander joins her colleagues in the ER to check on outside conditions, there is rain and howling wind. Because the storm had been downgraded when it made landfall, Olander now feels reassured. Her husband makes plans to return home, but she convinces him to stay until the next morning so they could leave together.

By that evening, they notice that most of the windows at the downtown Hyatt Hotel had been blown out:

"We were sitting by the pediatric emergency room outside on those cement benches. We could see the water starting to come this way. Initially we thought someone had turned on one of those fire hydrants. It wasn't this big gush of water. It wasn't on the sidewalk. It wasn't raining. I remember we sat out there that evening and it was twilight and we kept looking at the water. Where is this water coming from? But no one said anything, no big problems. We kind of buckled down for that evening and the first clue that things were not exactly as we thought was when an ambulance came up on the ramp. They had tried to get to Methodist Hospital and they got as far as right over the high-rise interstate ramp. . . . I don't think they got as far as Morrison Road in New Orleans East, because that is where the water was. One of the drivers was saying, 'We were trying to get to Methodist Hospital. They're underwater.' And we thought, 'Yeah, underwater, they don't want to take this patient they had in the ambulance.'"

Methodist Hospital is off Read Boulevard, and Olander's home is a few blocks away. "One of the drivers kept saying that at the Sam's and the Walmart, the water was at the roof of the Walmart. All you could see are the air-conditioning units and the top. He said there was an apartment complex at Interstate 10 and Crowder Boulevard. The water is past the first floor. Families are on the second floor, and the water is almost to the second floor."

It was then that the gravity of the news registers with her. "I had this horrible feeling, because I lived in the subdivision behind the Sam's. If there is water to the roof of Sam's, then my house is underwater. I remember I was crying. I never envisioned this. We never had water for the famous May 3 flood. I couldn't figure out where this water was coming from. That was Monday evening. Then we started getting patients from nursing homes. One of the questions was, 'Why are we getting patients from these nursing homes?' We thought they had plans that they were supposed to have in place. We were not talking about little old ladies, but were talking about vented patients."

From a nursing home in New Orleans East, Charity Hospital receives 10 patients on ventilators. At that point, there is still emergency power in the hospital. Later that evening, Olander returns to her office to try to get a few hours of sleep. A few hours earlier, the staff has successfully transferred an obstetric patient to University Hospital, but the water in the streets is slowly rising to sidewalk level. Tuesday, around 2:00 A.M., her supervisor, John, stationed at University Hospital, sends her a message. He said, "You need to move all the patients from the first floor as far up as you can. The 17th Street Canal has burst and the city is going to flood, and it is going to flood at a foot an hour." Olander adds, "That was the first time that I knew there was a major catastrophe."

When she returns to the ramp outside the ER, water completely covers the streets but had not yet reached the sidewalks. The staff starts moving patients. There are no elevators. In the basement, water already fills the cafeteria, the morgue, medical records, and dietary.

Patients who are not ambulatory are moved on stretchers. It requires six people to carry each patient to the second-floor auditorium. Olander says it was a monumental task. The staff also moves as much equipment and supplies as possible upstairs. On the second floor, they arrange some patients in the eye clinic, and the majority settle in the auditorium. Because they could not move all the patient beds, they bring mattresses to the auditorium on which to lay their patients.

"That was 6 days of backbreaking nursing care," she shares. "The nurses, they took care of those patients on the floor. We went to the various clinics looking for stretchers, but the problem is on the second floor. Those are more specialty clinics [few have beds]—eye clinic, dental clinic, so we didn't have exam tables or beds that we could put people on. The GI clinic on the second floor had stretchers, so we pulled those out and used them for some patients . . . but for the most part it was either that, a half an exam table, or chairs, so a good bit of the patients were on the floor. The auditorium was divided into one area for acute care patients, and another area for the less critical patients. There also were patients on ventilators. The hospital had six portable generators assigned to designated areas: one each for the emergency room, ICU, recovery, neuro ICU—and neuro ICU was full—SICU, MICU full, all of them were full. Recovery had the gunshot victim and the stabbing victim that had come in. So we divided up, and every area had one generator. One generator was needed for lights and for vents.

"Respiratory had activated respirators for their patients and used the E cylinders to power the respirators. Some patients needed to be hand-bagged for a while but were soon on generator-powered respirators.

"I have to say, I was really so proud of the staff because they were taking care of the patients like it was a normal day. They were turning them, keeping them clean. We had linen up to a point. Then we started going through all of the clinics and got linen wherever we could find it. We were pulling down supplies. Our warehouse was right down the street. Some of the maintenance people got the big truck and they would bring supplies. We had plenty of bottled water and we had to take some water to University Hospital because they were running out. The truck would bring supplies. We were overstocked on things that we never did need. We were well stocked on IV solutions and IV tubing. We needed more bed pans, practical stuff. More of those sterile bottles of water would have helped—1,000 cc bottles of water or saline would have helped—but, when I think about it now, we were well stocked for the worst major traumas to come in, and they didn't. But the truck made a couple of runs back and forth to the warehouse and I think that is how we got some food. The last time the truck came the water had gotten so high that it floated and crashed into one of the cars and a light post. Then the water got in the engine and it stalled. We couldn't use it anymore."

By Tuesday morning, the water begins creeping up the ER ramp. Cars parked on the street have water past their windows. Long corridors and stairwells are lit by flashlights. The heat rises to an unbearable 100° plus. Employees break windows to get air circulating in the hospital. From their vantage point on the ER ramp, Olander and her colleagues could see the lighted Veterans Administration Medical Center (VA) located across the street:

"And then an army truck arrived on the ramp with six vented patients. I asked why they did not bring them to the VA or check with other hospitals that had power. The army said, 'You take these patients.' It got to the point there was no arguing, so we took those patients. I asked our medical director of the emergency room, 'Have you called over at the VA and asked them could they possibly help us out?' We are getting patients in and we have no means of caring for them. It was not that we didn't want to care for them, but you're looking across the street and you see all these lights. Maybe we could get some of these patients over there. We'll send staff if that is the issue . . . eventually the CFO, COO, director of personnel, myself—there were about six of us—and we finally got one of them to listen. One of the doctors called the VA and they didn't know we had any problems . . . . The next time the army came, we told them the VA had power, and the army brought a couple of patients over there. We kept the ones that we had."

That evening, people who had taken shelter in their homes when the storm originally hit now seek shelter at Charity Hospital as the flooding worsened. They make their way along Tulane Avenue through waist-level, and sometimes chest-level, water. There are elderly and middle-aged people and parents with their young children. But by now, Charity Hospital has become a locked-down facility. Olander understands the necessity of lockdown. An influx of new patients will overburden the resources they have for their existing patients:

"We couldn't take anyone else. There was a limit to what we could do, but there were people that I saw, and I am talking old people, and I would think, 'Why can't we take this old lady? Just tell her children to go down to the Superdome' . . . it was like, 'We finally made it to Charity Hospital and they won't let us in.' It was really heartbreaking. We kept telling them to go to the Superdome. We would give them bottles of water and tell them go to the Superdome, never realizing the Superdome was having its horrendous problems."

Tuesday's meals, served in a Styrofoam cup for patients and staff, consist of canned mixed vegetables and sliced peaches. Breakfast, lunch, and dinner—the meal was the same. A find of canned chili was a welcomed dietary distraction. Olander says the staff was hopeful that evacuation was imminent, but when word circulates that CNN had reported that Charity Hospital was evacuated, morale plummeted.

That evening, the administrators receive notice that the National Guard is coming to evacuate the hospital. The task of readying the patients for the anticipated move proves to be frustrating, time consuming, and backbreaking. The plan is first to move the critical patients. Each patient's medical record is placed in a protective plastic sleeve, along with his or her medications.

"The National Guard didn't come. So we'd wake up the next morning and when we heard on the news that we had been evacuated, somebody got on their cell phone called wherever and said, 'No, we have not evacuated. We are still here. We have all of these patients. You need to come and get us.'" In attempts to combat low morale and quell rumors, Olander says administration holds meetings twice a day to explain to the staff that they are still in rescue mode, and efforts are directed to getting stranded residents off their rooftops before focusing on hospital evacuations. Olander's son Darryle, a New Orleans police officer, was scheduled to report to work on Tuesday morning for assignment in the Ninth Ward. When he got off work on Monday night, she convinced him to join his parents at the hospital.

"That meant he was stuck there, and there was no one to call. A lot of people who said that police left [didn't know] they were stuck in different places. I am eternally grateful I made my child stay with me, because he would have gone home and he would have drowned. He is such a hard sleeper. He would have been at home and drowned, gone to sleep and not awakened. But he was here with us. He worked with our hospital police in helping secure the hospital. One of the hospital housekeepers was hysterical. Her children were trapped in an attic with the babysitter. She came to work because she was required to come to work, but her children, thinking nothing was going to happen, were in the house with the babysitter. The only good saving thing was the cell phone. The babysitter called in said they were trapped in the attic . . . the person in charge of hospital police, my son, and a couple of other people went and they got those children out of there. And there were a couple of other people they rescued while they were in that building. But for the most part we kept hearing about people with guns who were raiding the hospitals for drugs. That did not happen. Most of that sensational stuff did not happen."

The medical staff navigates between Charity Hospital and University Hospital by boat. When they are told that Tulane Medical Center (located several blocks from Charity and University hospitals) was evacuating its patients, MCLNO negotiates to move some of the patients from Charity Hospital to Tulane. "It took six people to carry each patient. These were our physicians, our male nurses. We had some maintenance and dietary guys that were helping. They went up and down in the dark stairwells that were pitch black. We lit them with flashlights and started running out of batteries. We went up and down stairs. They got the patients over to Tulane and then there was this big snafu. Supposedly Tulane had evacuated all of their patients, but before they would take our patients they started evacuating their staff . . . and that is when we lost the patient staying on Tulane's roof overnight. . . . staff were irate, so after that we didn't send any more patients over to Tulane."

A low supply of diesel becomes another concern. Hospital staff raid the hospital's supply trucks for the precious fuel that power the generators. They siphon fuel from the ambulance parked on the ER ramp before the flood waters rise. Some doctors and nurses went to the Entergy Garage and siphoned diesel from cars and trucks. Generator use is limited at night. Staff store the newly acquired diesel fuel in garbage cans, gasoline cans, and 55-gallon drums. The eclectic collection of containers is placed on a corner of the ER ramp, under guard by the hospital police. Wednesday evening, an army jeep and truck drive up the ramp. A decorated soldier gets out of one vehicle and gets into the other. They leave.

Olander shakes her head. "We just sat there and looked at each other. We couldn't believe they did that in front of us—I don't know if they even knew the situation we were in, but to use our ramp to swap out vehicles—it was like they are not taking anybody. That was a blow. Wednesday, we are thinking, here comes the army to rescue us, and they brought us these patients. The next time they came with a big army diesel truck that brought us diesel fuel. It just arrived on the ER ramp. Whether it was supposed to come to us or not, we begged for the diesel and got it.

"By midweek, staff were taking turns showering. Once the flood reached the generators the [hospital] water went too; we didn't have pumps to get water. The commodes stopped flushing. . . . People would find a commode that hadn't been used and then all of a sudden word got out. By Wednesday people were cutting off the ends of their scrubs. I had brought with me two pairs of shorts and a tank top that was going to be my pajamas. But then that got to be work clothes . . . whatever made you comfortable, you wore it."

Efforts are made to make conditions as tolerable as possible for the patients. She adds, "The patients were very appreciative. They were thanking the nurses—we never had any arguments. We made sure every patient, if they could tolerate it, drank water at least every hour. We made sure they got their cup of vegetables, if they wanted it. Those who could walk we formed a little chain gang and would take them to the bathroom and try to keep them refreshed. We started using the sterile saline to freshen them up."

Staff are ready to prepare patients for transport on a moment's notice. Updates are given at morning and evening meetings in the lobby. "It was really getting to people—could see it was starting to take a toll by that Wednesday. It was hot, we had no food, but we had plenty of water. When we got diesel from the army, we told them we needed food and then we got the MREs [meals ready to eat]. They brought us boxes of rations so we could feed patients and staff. On Thursday, the hospital kept getting supplies, but what we needed was help evacuating our sick patients. Every day we got our patients ready for evacuation, but no help was coming. First it was to be the National Guard, and then it was the army, and later the navy. Every day we heard something different about who was coming to get us, and we would prepare the patients."

Thursday, a nurse's father arrives via boat to take his daughter out of the hospital. She won't leave. He is upset. The staff tells him no one was coming, and they have over 400 patients, family members, and employees to evacuate. The man says the news reported that they had evacuated. He promises that he and others would return the next morning to get everyone out. Olander has no way of knowing that this father whose call to a friend at the Louisiana Wildlife and Fisheries is the start of a rescue effort for her and the others at Charity.

"We said again, this is another promise. By that Thursday at the morning meeting, the staff was getting antsy. Our administration told the staff it was past rescue now—we had been told every day that the hospital was going to be evacuated, and every day nothing happened, so we just needed to be prepared, we might be here for another week or so. There was a prayer vigil out on the ramp, but the staff was starting to break down. Administration met with staff twice a day, in the morning, to let them know what happened overnight. We had gotten to the point where we had started packaging patients and bringing them down, and then they weren't going anywhere, so then the ER on the first floor started filling up with patients coming down. We were reusing the ER again mainly to staff patients from wherever they were coming from. That Thursday, we got more MREs; we still had plenty of water. We kept reminding staff to come down and get water. We had a line of people who were bringing water up to floors.

"We packed patients to be ready Thursday, and no one came . . . we had heard that message Tuesday, Wednesday, and Thursday, so we were thinking this is not going to happen. We had one of our doctors over in the Superdome. That is when we started hearing all of these horrible things going on in the Superdome. I recall when we had the teleconference that Monday when the storm first passes, with the Medical Center of Louisiana at New Orleans' chief executive officer. I told him, please talk to whomever you need to talk to. Don't let them open up the Superdome and let all of those patients come to us. We can't take it—I hope they have some plan to handle them in the Dome, because I could just see that happening—every day there were patients, there were people walking in that water, and the water had the oily horrible smell. I know there were bodies in that water. And I really believe that some of our homeless that lived around there died in that.

"We had one group of people that somehow made it up to the garage and it was a lady, an elderly diabetic, and her daughter and two little children. They made it up the stairs and they got to the garage where the garage meets the hospital, and they were banging on the doors, 'Please let us in!' We let her in—that lady would have died—she just needed to get in, but we kept all the doors closed and our hospital police maintained them. And what happened, usually at dusk when it started getting dark, one of the hospital police and one of the men, a hospital employee, each took a door and they manned the door and made sure that the doors were safe for the night. I can remember my son—going door to door—turned the ER doors off to close them.

"Charity Hospital had so many entrances—unbelievable, first and second floors. Doors that in the past you never thought about—those were the doors people were trying to get in. So we stationed someone who had a gun [an officer] and a regular employee, and they manned those doors from the evening until morning and usually during the day, but not with the same vigilance as at night.

"It was pretty much quiet at night. One of the things we didn't have was that roaming around—we told staff to stay where you needed to be. We definitely did not let visitors walk around. . . . There was an incident . . . supposedly there was shooting going on in Charity Hospital and the SWAT team landed on the roof or the 12th floor, and they came through the hospital. Where that rumor started I don't know. The SWAT team came through the hospital in the dark with their lights on. They found out nothing had happened and they left. The breaking-in to get narcotics did not happen.

"On that Thursday, we got some patients out in a refrigerator truck. Those were ambulatory patients—I don't know where they went. I don't know where they went to—initially the patients that went to Tulane Medical Center were accompanied by a nurse. If they were on a vent, they went with a nurse and a respiratory therapist. One had to come back because we were going to deplete ourselves of critical care nurses. For the most part the nurses stayed and respiratory came back.

"But the next morning, Friday, sure enough they had a line of those boats, like a flotilla out there to evacuate us. We talked to them about evacuating Charity Hospital, but University Hospital was in worse shape than us. We said go do University Hospital first. So they went to University Hospital. I thought they were not coming back. Thursday evening is when I really got depressed because we had moved some patients back and forth so many times, it was to the point where I didn't know how long these patients are going to make it.

"Thursday began on a high note when there was talk about evacuation. But that became another rumor. When Tulane did not take our patients and they took their staff instead, that was a blow. This time, we heard they didn't take our patients because someone was shooting at us. Now whether or not they were shooting at us, I don't know. You could hear periodic gunfire. People were saying they were not shooting at people; they were shooting to get attention. They didn't think anyone heard or saw them, so they shot . . . and it turned into a shooting match. I can say emphatically that none of that happened at Charity Hospital. No shooting, fighting, breaking in and stealing, or drug incidents occurred . . . all that crazy stuff did not happen at the hospital. I can honestly say I was never afraid of someone getting in here.

"I appreciated the way staff got together and manned the doors, too. To some extent, I felt in my heart we should have taken some people in, but I didn't have the authority to override administration. Some people walked from the Industrial Canal and made it to Charity Hospital. We have always been there for them and we didn't take them in. And that was difficult. By Thursday evening, you could tell people were really getting down. I had one nurse that totally flipped out. We had to send her up to the third floor [psychiatric unit] and give her some medication. She was one of the first ones we got out. For the most part, the nurses were just depressed, down. They continued to take care of their patients. I don't think any patient got a bedsore while they were there. They were kept dry and clean. We found linens. We had enough water. We had enough critical care supplies that we didn't need . . . we didn't need those extra IVs. We had plenty. If we were not rescued, I don't know how much longer the food and water would have lasted."

On Friday morning, relief finally comes to Charity Hospital. It is near 9:00 A.M., and it is from the Louisiana Wildlife and Fisheries. Patients, employees, and family members line up for evacuation. Most of the patients leave on airboats that take two at a time, loaded side by side in the hull. With no more spine boards, staff start taking doors apart. They also use privacy panels from the clinics.

"We took doors down and secured patients on doors. We carried patients from the 12th floor down. We got every patient downstairs. I was at the back door with one of our doctors. We listed every patient with their records. We didn't know where they were going. All we know is they were getting out of the hospital, taking them to the staging area for patients. I understand it was somewhere at Causeway, and some patients went directly to the airport. We were told we were going to go with our patients to either Dallas or San Antonio."

At her post, Olander writes in a tablet the name and medical record number of each patient before he or she left. They evacuate by air or boat. There were several ambulatory patients who are loaded into a military truck that sits high above the water.

"They looked like cattle, it was horrible to say, but they were sitting down in this big truck and where those people went to I don't know. If any critical patient left, a nurse went with them—it was determined that a nurse or a doctor went with them. Our doctor did not want any patient leaving us and going to a lesser area of care. The nurses packaged with each patient a week's supply of medicines along with their chart. Hopefully the patients were going somewhere they could get their medicines."

Evacuation takes all day Friday. After all the patients are evacuated, there remains a few dozen administrators. Staff makes a final sweep of each floor to make sure no one was left behind. Olander and her colleagues are taken by airboat to City Hall, where they board an air-conditioned charter bus.

"It was heaven to be on that bus," she says. "We left and went across the river because you couldn't get out of the city the other way. We crossed the river and came back to Interstate 10 to the airport. We got to Airline [Highway] right before you get to the airport. The Kenner Police stopped us. They got on the bus, rifles drawn, and asked us—I will never forget this—'Where the hell do you think you're going?' We said, 'We are from Charity Hospital, we are with our patients—we're supposed to go to the airport. A plane is going to take us to a hospital in either Dallas or San Antonio.'

"The police stated, 'I don't know who told you to do this.' Some of the doctors got up and spoke to the police. Then the police told us, 'Y'all go ahead, but there are no planes coming out of that airport.' The police let us go and our bus was back in line. There must have been hundreds of buses—school buses, regular buses—but we got separated from our patients.

"As we waited on the bus, some National Guardsmen with rifles drawn board the bus, telling us no one could leave. There were a few people milling around outside of their buses. We tried to explain we are supposed to be with our patients. We were told there are no patients; you have to stay. We left from one situation and were going to be sitting at this airport for days waiting to get out. The bus driver said he had come from Washington, D.C. He said he had two tanks full of gas and can take us wherever we want to go. His instructions were to evacuate people. We took a vote and everyone said let's go to Baton Rouge. The driver told the National Guardsmen that we wanted to get out of here and they let us back out, we made this tight turn and we left. We got on the interstate going to Baton Rouge.

"As we crossed over the Bonne Care Spillway near LaPlace, the driver said, 'I want you to look at something. Look over to your left. We have been sitting in that line of buses waiting for someone to tell us where to go and who to get. We have been sitting there for days, just waiting to go in to rescue.' I just got so full and tears were coming. There were double rows of buses lined up as far as you could see." The driver said they could get in, but no one was directing them, and they waited for days.

"No one coordinated or talked about how we were getting out. I could understand Monday or Tuesday they were rescuing people, and when you got down to Friday the Wildlife and Fisheries people were the ones who got us out. We didn't know where we were going, but the bus driver called Washington, D.C., and his contact called a church in D.C., who called a church in Baton Rouge. They told us that they would be glad to have us—so this bus took us to a church off Siegen Lane."

Olander's group arrives and are welcomed with a meal of red beans and rice and cots where they can sleep. Olander calls relatives who lived in Baton Rouge. They come to get her. She feels if it had not been for their bus separating from the others at the airport, they would have been in San Antonio where her colleagues had been sent.

On Tuesday, September 6, Olander goes to MCLNO's headquarters on Essen Lane in Baton Rouge to report for work. She sees a physician and asks what she needed to do. His reception is warm, and he directs her to the front desk. "He says, 'I am glad you're here. Go tell them at the desk you are here and who you are.' Maybe I was feeling the need for someone to take pity on me. The woman at the desk wrote my name and said, 'We'll be in touch with you.' I thought I was going to be working that day. The doctor had said, 'If nothing else, maybe you could talk to people who are calling.'" That was her dismissal.

Olander returns on Friday to see the hospital personnel director. She leaves and there is no call.

"The next thing we heard is they were going to start furloughing people; we were on paid leave until November. The administrator over ambulatory care had left a message on my answering machine asking where the list of patients that left the hospital was. When I left, I turned that over to either the COO or CFO. I gave the list away, and now they're calling me a week and a half later about what happened to the list. . . . Maybe it is still at Charity Hospital. That is the only call I got."

Olander is bitter having endured the 6 days at Charity Hospital, only to be released from work. She has lost her home, and now she has lost her job. After 35 years in nursing, maybe it is time to retire. She feels resentment because she was not in the planning discussions on the future of her department.

"I got very depressed because I had lost everything. I had lost my house, lost my job. We were staying with my husband's relatives—the best people in the world. They had just completed a mother-in-law's suite just off their house. Very nice. One bedroom, bathroom, and sitting area. We rented from them, so we did have some place to stay. We didn't lose any family members. And I started asking myself, 'Why are you so depressed? You have so much to be thankful for.'

"At the time, you could not tell me not to be so bitter. I had lost my house . . . and so I needed to be away. I was not going to get on any medication. Everyone jumps to some pill. I did not want this, but I did go see my doctor. It got to the point I was not getting up; I would stay in the bed all day.

"My husband went back to work. He would leave and I would lie down and look at movies, I got to the point where I just had to get out of bed. I realized then I was getting more depressed. I saw my physician, and she put me on something for a month. Then I started feeling better. I heard of people who were still looking for family members. All of my family had left. They were all safe. I had an aunt and cousin who didn't leave, and they were evacuated by helicopter, but they were safe. Lucky for us, we kept insurance up on my house and we had adequate flood insurance. Now when I think back, we had a lot to be thankful for.

"Maybe I needed to go back to work. We decided we were not coming back to our home. We built a house. That took some of my mind off of everything. I had told my director I looked forward to retirement and heard people say, 'Oh, you won't have anything to do,' and I thought, 'Let me just get to that point.'"

In January 2007, Olander returns to work. She works part-time as an Angel of Mercy—a core of nurses, including retired ones, who serve as patient liaisons for the ER. They communicate between the medical staff and the patients' family members and are there to offer consolation. It is a program she began several years ago at Charity Hospital. She commutes from her home in Prairieville, between Baton Rouge and New Orleans. Renovations on her former home in New Orleans East should be completed in 2009.

Four years post–Hurricane Katrina, memories of Charity are always close. "I am still amazed at the selfless dedication of the staff. It was 6 days of hell. It was unbelievable. For 6 days staff cared for patients on their knees, giving IVs, giving medications, turning, cleaning patients on their knees. We were in it together and everyone worked there as a team.

"Patients—you would always hear the staff say the patients don't care. But oh, they do care. They are appreciative. The problem is you don't listen. You don't listen to what they're telling you. You are assuming they have a complaint or whatever and all they want to do is say thank you, or 'I appreciate it,' and they did. Our patients were very appreciative. I just wonder why we didn't get some of those people out of the city even if we didn't think the worst was going to happen. There was no reason that those nursing home patients weren't evacuated to someplace. The electricity was going to go off—how were you going to maintain the vents? You didn't have generators, forget the water—you were not going to be able to maintain them.

"I was one of the staff members for Charity Hospital that worked with the city on evacuation planning. The city was going to use the Superdome for special needs. I was in a meeting where the city officials talked about the possibility of a mandatory evacuation, and I said to someone next to me, 'What does that mean?' You have a city where more than half the population relies on public transportation, and you are going to issue the order to evacuate people who do not have a car, and drive to a hotel that they don't have money to pay for, and just sit there when they are living day to day on assistance or without public transportation. I never could understand why we didn't have staging areas to take them out in buses. They were very arrogant, with the attitude 'we can't be all things to all people' . . . but at some point in time you know that your city's population relies on public transportation. . . . Why then would you not have that public transportation to get them out of here?

"The staff went above and beyond. A lot of people did not realize what really went on in these hospitals and what staff had to deal with. I was very proud that we took care of our patients, and our goal was, everyone is getting out. However we did it, we were going to do the best that we could, and staff was behind it 100%."

Andrea Adams

Everything I have learned about evacuation for patients, I learned from Katrina.

Andrea Adams, RN, started her psychiatric nursing career in 1970 as a licensed practical nurse and has been working in psychiatry ever since. She received a registered nurse diploma in 1978 from Methodist School of Nursing in her hometown of Memphis, Tennessee, and received her

BSN from Loyola University in New Orleans in 1991. She has worked for 39 years in the specialty of psychiatry and has held various roles such as staff nurse, educator, and administrator. She started working at Charity Hospital in August 1997, as the associate nurse administrator, up until Katrina. Post-Katrina she has the privilege of working at the renowned Menniger Clinic, now located in Houston, "before returning to New Orleans and my previous employer, now known as Interim LSU Public Hospital."

August 28, 2008, on the third floor of Charity Hospital's psychiatric unit, Andrea has 98 patients under her watch. Her staff are assigned 12-hour shifts; they make sure medications are given without interruption and have soft music playing throughout the five units. In addition to her staff, there are 42 family members of patients and employees.

The heat, and each day passing with the unfulfilled promise of imminent evacuation, begins to wear on her staff. There are reports of snipers outside, and the nurses move the patients away from windows and into the hallways. Periodic breaking of windows signal someone's attempt to encourage air circulation in the hospital. The sounds of helicopters can be heard as stranded residents are plucked from rooftops. "It felt like a war zone. It was a traumatic experience," she adds.

"As the nurse administrator, I felt like the captain of my ship. . . . When I walked the units, no lights, no air-conditioning, there was such calm. It was eerie how quiet it was. We would take our patients out of their rooms. Every morning we would brief our staff and have an opening prayer. It is amazing that in adverse conditions, how people pull it together. We worked in sync. Even with our patients—they know fear, and they seek those who they trust."

Reports about the storm and the wake of its path filter to her via news media reports. To her dismay, the reports are not always accurate.

"They were not in the hospital. They did not know what people were going through minute by minute. By the grace of God we were faced with a national disaster. Just the story of the human spirit in a disaster was incredible. Through times like that we are trying to work as one. We were all survivors."

By chance, she has phone contact with two nurses in Florida, who call her during the 6-day stay at Charity Hospital. Andrea does not know how they reached her, but they became her "lifeline." On the fifth day, when Andrea and her colleagues are told there is no definitive timeline for evacuation, Andrea cries. She could not bear to tell her staff to wait one more day.

But evacuation comes the next day, when they put their patients on a military truck. They are taken to the Superdome, where they are transferred to buses. She stays in Pineville for a week and then heads to Memphis to be with her family and friends. A few days later, an emotionally and physically exhausted Andrea starts crying and has difficulty stopping. She reunites with her 17- and 21-year-old daughters, who had evacuated to Houston, where all three of them begin counseling. Her home in New Orleans was destroyed by nearly 5 feet of water, but Andrea saved what was most important to her—family photographs.

Katrina taught her lessons in evacuation. "Everything I have learned about evacuation for patients, I learned from Katrina: having those large lanterns; the importance to organize; knowing your patients and your staff. Not everyone can be on the evacuation team. There was staff we had to pull off. You have to know what stresses are in a person's life."

On September 25, 2007, officials from the Interim LSU Public Hospital opened a 33-bed hospital psychiatric care unit in the Seaton Building at the former DePaul Hospital. The campus at 1035 Calhoun Street is nestled in the residential area of Uptown New Orleans, near Audubon Park and the Mississippi River. Andrea calls it the perfect location for a mental health facility, surrounded by majestic oaks and open green spaces for the patients. In her capacity as head nurse manager, and with limited personnel, Andrea helped to open the unit. She wrote all the policies and procedures and even retrieved furniture from the shuttered Charity Hospital. Looking out from the second-floor window in the conference room near her new office, Andrea calls nursing "my purpose in life. I get so much joy working with patients."

John Jones

The flooding caused us the problems, otherwise we would have defended in place, the way we had always done. We didn't evacuate anybody. We have learned from that experience.

John Jones, RN, MN, NEA-BC, had been employed at MCLNO (Charity and University hospitals) for 16 years. Prior to his retirement in August 2009, John was the chief nursing officer at MCLNO. He had experience in a variety of leadership and administrative positions in New Orleans and Florida over the past 43 years. Raised in Fort Lauderdale, Florida, hurricane season was part of life.

Storms came with the territory for John. When he reports to work at 7:00 A.M. for his post as associate administrator of patient care services, Hurricane Katrina is less than 24 hours to landfall. His only sense that this storm is different from previous ones is when he sees its massive size on news reports. Its sustained winds reach 175 mph and extend 120 miles from its center. If he had not been scheduled for work that day, he would have considered leaving town, something he had never done when other hurricanes threatened the area.

Collectively, the medical campuses of Charity and University hospitals have a patient census of 400 and close to 1,000 staff to ensure around-the-clock coverage. That number does not include family members unreported by employees. Spouses and children go unnoticed when administrators make their rounds. When it is time to evacuate, the tally of evacuees rise with these uncounted persons. At Charity and University hospitals, inventories for linens, pharmaceuticals, food, and water are stocked to provide for 2 weeks of provisions. "The truth is we didn't run out of anything," observes John. "We did not have tap water because electrical power had been cut, and running water had stopped functioning. The electricity went out. In terms of water to drink and food, there were no shortages.

"Communications initially were fine because we had everything functioning. As the flooding occurred, the phone lines were underground, and we lost phones. The towers blew off and the cells phones weren't reliable. They lasted as long as the battery did, but it was nearly impossible to get a line through anyway. You could text, but phone lines were impossible. We had one generator with bunches of cell phones hooked up to it. A satellite phone allowed minimal outside contact." Although he describes external communications as awful, there were two phones that are operational after the power failure. One is at the medical office building across the street from University Hospital, and another is in the back office. "The phones could only be used for outgoing long-distance calls. A phone line would go silent before you finished dialing.

"Nobody yet has been able to explain to me why these two phones continued to work, but I called my sister in Ft. Lauderdale and I said, 'Tape CNN for me, because we don't have any power, I can't see what's going on, and tell everybody I am all right and that's all I am saying, because there is a whole line of people that want to get to this phone,'" he recalls. The fragmented internal communications were a challenge when John hears early Tuesday that the levees have failed and the city is flooding. It is 2:00 A.M., and he needs to reach Olander Holloway on the Charity campus. He cannot assume they have received the same message. After much effort, he finally reaches Mary and tells her that vertical evacuation is activated and to move patients to the second floor.

"And once I reached Mary, who was one of Olander's right hands, then I knew it was taken care of and I could quit worrying about them getting notified. I knew they had been informed because Mary, if she had to carry a lantern through every building to let every person know, she would."

Floodwaters come into Charity Hospital's basement, and at University Hospital, the water pours into the loading dock. Despite the closing of the dock's floodgates, the water cannot be stopped. The staff knows it is only a matter of time until power would go down. Generators are set up in all critical care areas. There are no patient transfers. "We were defending in place," John explains. "Had the levees not broken and had we not flooded, we would have gone through this storm like we did every other hurricane. In fact, I looked out the window of my office and I could see a truck parked across the street. Water was up to the running board, and I would gauge the level of flooding, and think, 'OK, I guess we'll sleep here tonight and tomorrow, and then we can go home.' Like we had many times before, I went to sleep, and when I got up the floodwater was up to the truck's window. The flooding caused us the problems, otherwise we would have defended in place the way we had always done. We didn't evacuate anybody. We have learned from that experience."

When a woman arrives in labor, delivery of the baby by cesarean section seems likely. However, it is not needed. Mom and new baby are readied for air evacuation. John recounts, "When the babies were carried to Tulane Hospital's parking garage, where they went up to the roof, they got stopped. They stopped the [NICU] babies, too. They had to bring them back over to Charity Hospital and kept them there until we could get them out. Finally, we got word that our babies were going to be taken out to a children's hospital in Shreveport by helicopter.

"The thing that also impressed me was this: Even though, after the city flooded, staff knew they lived in an area like New Orleans East and that their home was underwater, but that was something they had to shove to a compartment in the back of their brain because there was nothing they could do about it. They had patients to take care of. There were a couple of people who were affected by the storm and the conditions in the building for that long—who were acting erratic—and we had to take them out of patient care and let them rest, give them some intravenous fluids, but that was two or three—very limited. What is important is to keep your eye on what is going on with what the people are doing, because stress doesn't necessarily show up the same in all people. By observing behavior, you can spot that something is not right.

"When the National Guardsmen brought a group of patients from a nursing home, our staff told them their resources were maxed and they were not a shelter. They set them in the parking lot and said, 'Well, you can just leave them there,' and left. And so of course, we didn't leave them in the parking lot. They were people who had severe physical and mental impairments—some were children—so we brought them inside and took care of them.

"I am really very proud of everybody and the work that they did. I don't think that anybody stumbled. I am proud of how they conducted themselves during that entire time. There were only two incidents that concerned me, that really frightened me. In the middle of the night, six boats arrived with maybe a dozen plus officers. They came to secure a prisoner patient that we had. That patient was in the intensive care unit, seriously ill, and wasn't going to do anything to anybody, but he was a prisoner patient and the police officers came to take him back. They arrived with their guns . . . like one of those raids in Entebbe. They came and got the guy, put him in a boat and off they went.

"That didn't frighten me, in a sense of personal danger, but this is scary. What kind of patient do we have here that you come and do this in the middle of the night? I think it was more of the police's overreaction than anything else. The guy was ill and he wasn't going to cause any kind of problems. However, he was secured by agents of the appropriate authority."

The second incident involved five young men who were floating in a hot tub, "who were obviously up to no good, having a grand time coming to the hospital to get drugs," says John. "I was dismayed at the ladies up on the crosswalk egging them on. And as I looked down on the crosswalk, our [University Hospital] security was standing on the emergency room ramp with their guns and said, 'If you want to get shot, this is the right place to be—come on.' And the guys' egos wouldn't allow them to paddle backward, but they quit paddling and the current let them drift back around the corner. But those five men were up to something. If they had come into the building, there would have been problems. Our hospital security stopped them—it was frightening to watch that. In the middle of all of this mess that we're in, there are people doing that kind of stuff."

John says no one was cavalier about their duties. "We were prepared for the storm, but not prepared for the flooding. The flooding was a blessing in that it kept a lot of people away from us. Like the guys in the hot tub. If we had not had the flooding, who knows who would have been coming in what door or where. It was like a moat around both Charity and University hospitals that kept away stuff we didn't need to deal with."

The several false calls about evacuation become wearisome for him and his colleagues. His sister tells him the media has reported that MCLNO was cleared of all personnel and patients. He tells her they had it wrong. Having served in the navy, John says orders are followed, not debated. "When you are given an order, you don't sit there and say, 'Oh, they're shooting guns,' or 'Oh, the water is too deep.' When you are given an order, you move! Our government simply did not give the military the order to do something for far too long. We were in there far too long. . . . I can see where they were using their resources to rescue people from rooftops, and I can forgive them for that because we were, even though we were sweaty and hot, in a safe place.

"But at night, watching the platoons come in across Interstate 10—it's like they were given the order to come in now, because here they come—why it took that long for them to get us out I don't know. To me that was a really negative, a negative taste that I have. The order to evacuate us should have come much sooner. It was as if everybody sat around deciding who they could point their fingers at."

He is not concerned about their supplies or their safety. Despite the physical labor, the hospital is secure. "If we needed to stay here another day, we stay here another day. I chanted silently a whole lot that, too, 'This too shall pass.' I didn't do it out loud. I just sat there and sweated and told myself this will be over; it will end. I am pretty stoic when it comes to that kind of stuff. I knew ultimately that we would get out of there. How long 'ultimately' was, I didn't know. I never had concerns about us not getting out. If need be, we would have floated on doors. Heat and taking the stairs—8 flights at University Hospital, 12 at Charity Hospital—proved physically challenging for everyone."

John describes Friday's evacuation of patients and staff as extraordinarily impressive. "Helicopters used the fifth-floor roof and the hospital roof as heliports. When one of the pilots walked into the Incident Command Center and announced that he had landed and our roof was soggy, the response from the group was one of bafflement." A continuous flow of airboats ferry patients and employees away to staging areas for evacuation from the city. As soon as a boat leaves the ER ramp with its passengers, another one takes its place. No one knows their final destination. No one can tell John and his colleagues where they are taking the patients. John's is among the last group to evacuate. They are taken to Loyola Avenue and board buses. Again, John said there is no word where they were going. They arrive at Louis Armstrong International Airport.

"At the airport, one of the things that will always haunt me is this poor lady from a nursing home who was obviously senile. There was a bunch of people from a nursing home. They were scared to death. I wanted so much to say to her, 'You're OK, you are going to be all right,' but I didn't have a lot of reserve left at that point and if I say anything to her she is going to come over here and lean on me and I have enough to deal with. So I just kept in the line and I still regret that I didn't have more reserve to do something more for that lady because she looked so lost and absolutely terrified."

John is one among thousands of evacuees at the airport. After standing in line for 2 hours, he reaches the information desk, where he gives his name and social security number. He boards a C130, not aware that the plane is going to San Antonio Air Force Base. There he reconnects with three colleagues. They leave the processing line and take a cab to the Riverside Hilton for a one-night stay. The next morning, they rent a car with plans to reach Houston later that day. When they stop for a meal, strangers next to their table pay their restaurant tab, having heard they are New Orleans evacuees. By the time they reach Houston, there is only John and another colleague. The other two earlier reunite with their families. In Lake Charles, Louisiana, John drops off his colleague and drives to Baton Rouge. It is the closest he could get to New Orleans. He returns to Houston and buys a one-way ticket to Atlanta, where his brother lives.

Talking about the post-traumatic stress that he saw impact people working in the city, including himself, he says, "You learn to deal with what you have to deal with . . . to go to the grocery store. Now I drive across town because the grocery store three blocks from home has no roof on it. So I think that we minimize those kinds of things that we have to adapt to, but they affect us."

With Charity and University hospitals out of commission, medical services resume in a tent city located in the parking lot next to University Hospital. Operations move into the New Orleans Convention Center. They later relocate to the vacant Lord and Taylor on Poydras Street.

In April 2006, the Elmwood Medical Center is leased for Charity's trauma services. The following year, trauma services return to University Hospital.

The hospital workforce became a casualty of the storm—a layoff that impacts the 4,000 employees who were kept on the payroll through December 2005. Notes John, "The system reaches a point that it doesn't have the resources and so laying off 4,000 people that you worked with for 20 or 10 years, or 5, and then bringing them back up, was a challenge by itself. Under civil service rules [you] have to bring back employees by seniority. Fortunately, civil service agreed that competence factored into who would return, so if the most senior person was a neonatal intensive care nurse, and if you didn't have that service, you could skip over that person. So it became a challenge to review clinical experience and work with civil service rules—this person's history and this one's competence—to see who was the right person to bring back to work . . . all of that taxed our energies."

For emergency preparedness, he advises, "Be reasonable and be prepared, but don't be overreactive. I still have this resentment about the media and about every storm coming. . . . I realize they can't ignore it, but the way they hype it up sounds like you can't get worse than that. So, you alarm people.

"People who go into nursing are committed to nursing, and when something happens they are committed to being there. If it is a fire, or earthquake, whatever, nurses are going to be there doing what they need to do to take care of patients. The whole profession is so dedicated, it's amazing. If there is a need, here we come. We will be the first ones there and the last ones to leave. Just recently, the Gallup Poll voted nurses the most reliable, and the most trusted, and nursing has earned that."

Marie May Traylor

I can't believe this was happening. It was extremely bad. It was just amazing. . . . Some people are blocking it out. I am guilty of that. When people ask me about it, I still can't comprehend every nuance, every little thing, every quiet heroic thing that transpired.

Marie May Traylor, RN, graduated from Touro Infirmary in 1979. She has worked in oncology and worked at Charity for many years in the postanesthesia care unit. She is currently working at Interim LSU Public

Hospital. She has been married for 29 years and has three children and one grandchild. She continues to learn something new every day, and she says she has "not lost my enthusiasm for my profession."

Since her first day on the job in 1981 as a Charity Hospital nurse, Marie May Traylor worked shifts in the recovery room on the 12th floor of the hospital. Later, she switched to working nights and weekends. Recovery is a sister unit to the intensive care unit. The nursing staff is cross-trained to draw support from each other, as needed. When she arrives at work that Sunday, August 28, there is one patient in recovery. Marie is one of six nurses in the unit. Across the hall, the ICU is full with 12 patients. Because the daily briefings are on the first floor, Marie says her floor was isolated from regular communications. Cell phones do not work, but a colleague's office has a WATS (wide area telephone service, used for long-distance calls) line receiving incoming calls.

Tuesday, the hospital loses power. Portable generators are carried up several flights of stairs to recovery. Later, when they have to switch to the ambu-bags for their ventilator-dependent patients, the staff hand-bag the patients up to an hour during the transition period. They use wet towels and ice packs, while they last, to cool the patients in the stifling heat of the hospital. The nurses' sleeping quarters are in the isolation room. Following her shift, Marie tries to sleep during the day, but it is difficult amid the noise of fellow nurses breaking windows in their attempts to cross-ventilate the patient care areas. Some of her colleagues go to the first floor, where administration gives daily communications briefings, but she does not leave her unit.

"I am kind of like that," she says. "I am going to stay with the core group. I am not going off on my own. When my sisters called and said they'll come get me, I am like, 'No, I am fine. Don't come anywhere near this place.'"

By the middle of the week, fatigue, sleep deprivation, and the heat take their toll on the staff. Communications are fractured. The nurses stay away from windows in case someone decides to shoot at the building. Deceased patients are placed in an open stairwell. A nurse on the fourth floor is admitted to the psychiatric unit.

"One of our nurses almost got in a fistfight with this doctor because he would come up and give us reports so dramatic, and paint such a dark picture, that the younger nurses were getting upset. This older male nurse said, 'Get the hell out of here, we don't need the drama with the information,'" Marie shares. She says her colleagues helped her cope during the 6 days they were at Charity Hospital following Hurricane

Katrina. "The people worked because they were just a great support system," she offers. "When I was feeling blue, they would tease me or do something to cheer me. We all worked together. There is nobody doing it for you. They were making it airier. The guys were making it secure . . . were locking up other units. Our housekeepers kept our bathrooms clean. We had an increased number of people using the bathrooms, and our housekeepers continued cleaning. They were amazing.

"We had a wonderful nursing assistant who had a sister on the 8th floor, so he would go from the 12th to the 8th floors and check on his sister. And then he would go from 8 to 6, where the cafeteria had moved. He would pick up whatever they were serving and bring it back to 12. It was our people that made that happen and made it as bearable a situation as it could be," she adds.

At her home in the Mid-City area of New Orleans, her husband and their two sons weather the storm. The flooding stops at the front steps to the house. On Tuesday, she loses contact with her family. The uncertainty about their safety is difficult for Marie, but she focuses on work. There are patients to care for.

Marie's voice waivers. "That was just really hard, because you don't know what is going on and some people don't have family in the city, so they are doing better. It's just that certain parts of the week I was doing better. I always say this. I wasn't the best employee. I wasn't the worst. I had my ups and downs. I was worried about what was going on because we would hear stories of looting and shootings. Some of my coworkers were shot at when they were transporting patients to Tulane's roof. We don't have guns. We are in the heart of the city. I guess people were running amok. People started coming to the Superdome, and you could see all of those poor people. . . . We could see a serpentine line and see the helicopters. And we heard horror stories about what was happening at the Superdome. It was so hot."

On Thursday, September 1, Marie receives word that her husband has rescued her 90-year-old mother from her Park Esplanade apartment that fronts Bayou St. John, across from City Park and the New Orleans Museum of Art. She had assumed her mother had left the city before the storm but learns later that her daughter had stayed with her mother in a first-floor apartment. As water began seeping into the apartment complex, the residents were moved upstairs. When Federal Emergency Management Agency (FEMA) personnel came to evacuate the residents to the Superdome, Marie's daughter refused to let them take her grandmother.

The next day, Marie's sister arrives from Dallas. With her is her nephew, a sharpshooter for the Dallas police, and Marie's brother-in-law. The armed trio rendezvous with one of her brothers, who brings a boat from Baton Rouge. It will be needed to reach her mother's apartment complex. They return to Dallas with her mother.

Also, on that Thursday the 12th-floor hospital staff prepare their patients for evacuation. They place them on stretchers and begin the slow descent down the stairs. They use the outside stairwells to take advantage of the daylight. Nurses, physicians, and medical students help with the task. They hand-bag their ventilator-dependent patients, maintaining the same rate as when they were on the ventilator. When they reach the first floor, they follow a hallway connected to the ER. From there, boats take them from the hospital to a staging area.

Marie says she and her coworkers were removed from day-to-day communications from administration during those days at Charity Hospital. On Friday, September 2, Marie gets in line to wait her turn to leave the hospital. She sees patients in the hallway. They, too, are waiting to leave.

"That was bad," says Marie. "We are all ready with our bags, whatever you could take, and there are still poor patients in the hallway. I remember one lady on a stretcher. She said, 'Oh, I am so thirsty.' I gave her some water, got her a cool rag."

By boat, Marie and her colleagues are brought to Loyola Avenue, where they are deposited one block from City Hall. The area is busy with a continuous stream of Wildlife and Fisheries boats unloading passengers, who then board school buses. Marie boards a bus that goes to Louis Armstrong International Airport. The bus driver has come from Arkansas. Her fellow passengers are patients and staff from the hospitals. En route to the airport, she learns that one of the hospital physicians on the bus has arranged for a private plane to take his staff from New Orleans. At the airport, eight passengers disembark from the bus. From her bus seat, Marie silently watches crowds of people. Several people move toward the bus.

"They wanted to get on the bus. I don't know what the purpose was of the airport. It was very sad," she relates. "After that sidetrack we get back in the queue with all the buses and we don't know where we're going. Nobody knows. There is no direction. And it is getting late at night, because my bus left around five. It is almost nine o'clock. We are still on Airline Highway by the airport. We are at a standstill for hours and hours. No directions. Nobody prepared for when we did get on the bus. Maybe they were utilizing that time to prepare. We finally go west. It took us 7–9 hours to complete this trip, from 5:00 to around 2:00 A.M., just to reach Baton Rouge. But there is no traffic. Traffic is not the issue."

Exhausted, she arrives at a reception hall that is filled with several evacuees. She contacts a niece who lives nearby. Within hours, Marie is at her niece's home, where 14 of her niece's friends have taken shelter. The next morning, with a one-way ticket and no other possessions, Marie takes a flight to Dallas. She remains there for 8 months at her sister's home. Marie's youngest son stays with her. The rest of her family is scattered. Her daughter is in college. Another son heads to Virginia. Three weeks after the hurricane, her husband returns home to resume work. Marie takes her retirement money, pays off debt, and plans for her family to have a one-salary income. Returning to nursing is not in her plans. On April 24, 2006, the LSU Health Care Services Division, MCLNO, reopens its Trauma Care Center at its temporary location in Jefferson Parish. Marie is offered a job there. She declines.

"They wouldn't guarantee any kind of hours and no kind of seniority mattered. And then I met a few of my former coworkers at the mall. They said, 'Come back'; I was hired without a job interview."

In February 2007, she returns to nursing. She says those 6 days at Charity Hospital probably read "like a fairy story. I can't believe this was happening. It was extremely bad. It was just amazing. . . . Some people are blocking it out. I am guilty of that. When people ask me about it, I still can't comprehend every nuance, every little thing, every quiet heroic thing that transpired.

"I have a friend, Debbie, who was great the whole time we were at the hospital. . . . She brought two ice chests full of stuff, and when we are feeling low Debbie breaks out a fresh pineapple. That's amazing to me. Who would think to bring a fresh pineapple? And then my other friend Ann lives in LaPlace and has two small children and an elderly mom. She never cried. She would tell me, 'Oh, Marie you're going to be fine. Your family is going to be fine. The Lord says they all will be fine.' Do you know when she cried?" Marie's eyes mist. "She cried when she told me good-bye! And she never cried the whole time. We worked every weekend together.

"I think that we would love to be back where we were, love to be back at Charity, to everything the way it was. I really do," she continues. "But has it been good in respect to a lot of people? I'd say that is has. One friend got a great job with the Department of Health and Human

Services. She critiques hospitals. My friend is now a supervisor. Different things for different people. We were compensated, but one of the things I was really upset and angry about is that not one of the supervisors called and said, 'Marie, thanks for doing a good job.' One supervisor I had known for 25 years. No thanks for staying till the end. 'Appreciate it. How are you doing now?' Nobody called. I myself would try to call. Nobody from the supervisory level would call at all.

"I don't think about Charity Hospital too much because my experience was not as bad as others.' . . . I always do that to myself—nurses do that," she says, "and I had a better outcome, so I don't think about it too much. Have you ever read *The Purpose-Driven Life*? You are always waiting for something kind of big to come along and say, 'This is it,' but maybe it is just being kind to a patient and helping them a little bit each day." She pauses. "My story is neither the biggest nor the best, but it is mine."

Gail Gibson

Let's just try to control what we can control. Take care of ourselves number one, and then we can take care of the patients.

Gail Gibson, RN, MN, graduated from LSU Medical Center in 1985 with a BSN and a master of science degree in nursing in 1994, with a focus in maternal–child health and nursing administration. She has been a nurse for 25 years. Gail is currently working at Medical Center of Louisiana at New Orleans (University Hospital) as the nurse administrator for labor and delivery. She has worked at MCLNO for over 20 years in various positions.

KATRINA STILL POWERFUL BUT GRADUALLY WEAKENING AS IT MOVES FARTHER INLAND. A HURRICANE WARNING IS IN EFFECT FOR THE NORTH CENTRAL GULF COAST FROM MORGAN CITY LOUISIANA EASTWARD TO THE ALABAMA/FLORIDA BORDER . . . INCLUDING THE CITY OF NEW ORLEANS AND LAKE PONTCHARTRAIN. (National Hurricane Center, 2005b)

The storm roars through New Orleans. At the Incident Command Center on the fourth floor at University Hospital, administrators feel assured that another bullet has been dodged. It is Monday, August 29, and they are assessing storm damage and determining when the first round of employees should be released from work. Their planning is interrupted when a hospital security officer runs into the boardroom shouting that the water was rising. Gail Gibson says that the group is stunned by the news. There is no rain. The storm had passed. Then the officer says it is rising quickly. The group runs downstairs. Outside, on the ER ramp, they see water creeping up from the street.

University Hospital had recently hired a licensed ham radio operator. He is helpful, but the communications from outside are sporadic. Not knowing when the water would stop rising, patients and supplies are moved from the first floor. Four critically ill patients remain there with assigned staff. The physicians are reluctant to move these frail patients, as they are on ventilators. The decision is made to keep them on the first floor until they absolutely have to be moved. Gail says they were "blessed the water did not come that high."

Gail had worked in the women's unit at MCLNO for 20 years. She was on staff at Charity Hospital and returned to University Hospital's maternal–child services. For several years, when code gray (the code to

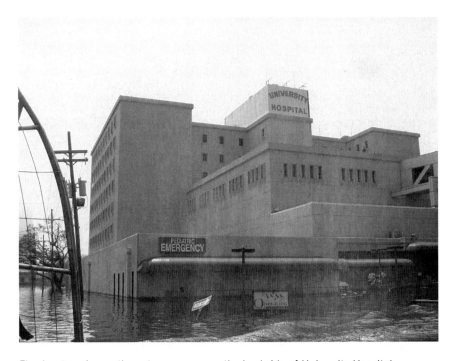

Flood waters rise up the entrance ramp on the backside of University Hospital.

alert staff to prepare for an impending hurricane) was activated before a storm, a satellite delivery and nursery nursing staff was set up at Charity, their sister hospital. The satellite had not been needed for previous storms, but for Hurricane Katrina, it was needed and used.

There are five deliveries during that week, with two at Charity Hospital. The last baby arrives Thursday night. It is a 23-week-old preemie whose delivery the nursing staff had tried to delay until they could evacuate her mother. Generators are set up on every floor that had any equipment on emergency power. For Gail's unit, there are two—one in delivery and one in the nursery. When the equipment is tested before the baby's delivery, the staff realizes they need more than one generator. "We used two generators in the operating room to deliver and then wound up having to use about three to keep all of the equipment going for the baby. The baby was a little one—one of the first ones to go when we started transferring folks out. We got that baby out fast."

On Wednesday, Gail says, they are informed that a helicopter evacuation is planned. The obstetric nurses would be ferried by rowboats to Tulane, three blocks away. In their arms, each nurse carries a newborn. A respiratory therapist accompanies the entourage. One baby is on a ventilator, and during the transport, the respiratory therapist hand-bags the newborn—forcing air into the tiny patient's lungs.

But the evacuation never happens. They return to University Hospital in tears. They had been told their patients could not be taken, as Tulane is doing its last evacuation of personnel and family members. "Oh, that was probably one of the roughest times," says Gail. "They came in, they were crying, they were angry, they were upset. They got off the boat. I pulled them into the waiting room because our boat dock was right in back of the hospital. I told them the important thing is that they made it back, they're safe, the babies are safe, bring the babies back up, get them settled and taken care of and we'll find out what the next steps are.

"They were extremely upset, and we talked about controlling the things you can. And what we had to control right now is making sure the moms stay calm and the babies were taken care of. I told them they were doing a great job at that and we'll go back and worry about the rest of the stuff. And that is kind of pretty much how we handled that.

"We had one nurse who was just so emotionally drained and upset that I told her, 'Look, you don't have to go on the transport the next time,' and she was like, 'No, I want to do it, I want to do it. I am just going to go and take a break.' It was very difficult. They thought they had got to the point where they were going to get the babies out, and it didn't happen."

Keeping communications flowing to the nurses is critical. Gail makes rounds two, sometimes three times a day to every unit, covering eight floors. When there is word about the breaks in the levees, many employees become anxious. Some visitors become restless.

"It was a handful dealing with some family members. We never ran out of food, but we had to ration. They thought that the staff had some special little dining area, having steak and potatoes, and we were giving them a little bowl of applesauce or something. The kitchen was downstairs and we had to move it upstairs. Whatever we could carry up, that's what was saved and that's when we started to ration food. We had so many people in-house. We had to feed patients—that was our priority." Not all visitors had brought their own supply of food. Some got angry with the meager rations. "Or they wanted a bed and there were no beds," recounts Gail. "They really got angry. At one point, the first day, the National Guardsmen had to come and get some visitors out who were threatening staff. These visitors were angry because they thought that we had more than what we had. We are eating the same thing. We get the same amount of water."

The unruly visitors are taken to the Superdome, where over 20,000 have taken shelter. Across the street from the hospital, on the fourth floor of a medical office building, someone discovers a working phone. Arrangements are made for employees to take turns for a 5-minute phone call to their loved ones. After 24 hours of connecting employees to the working phone, administration shuts the line down when security concerns arise. People from the neighborhood are trying to get into the building.

For Gail, her major and most time-consuming work is keeping the communications lines open to her staff. With some, she has to sit alone with them and talk or pray. She listens as they share their anguish about not knowing how their family is. She reminds them that their first priority is to take care of themselves so they can take care of their patients.

"If you're a basket case, you're not going to be able to be with them when you get out of there because you're going to be sick or need help, so let's just try to control what we can control. Take care of ourselves number one, and then we can take care of the patients," she says.

"[I kept] trying to keep them focused and to have some optimism that things are not only going to work out for us and the patients, it's going to work out for our family members and they're going to be happy to see the smiles on our faces when we get out of here and get to go and see them."

Before she was activated to work for the storm, Gail brought her two daughters, ages 17 and 6, to their grandmother's in Baton Rouge. Her husband, a pharmacist, was tending to last-minute requests from patrons of his home infusion business. He said he might ride out the storm at the family's home on the West Bank. Gail told him that would not be a good idea. Her mother and sisters had opted to stay at the Hilton Hotel on Canal Street, near the Mississippi River, where her brother-in-law was a manager. By Monday, they were part of the hotel's mass exodus when the waters began rising. She does not learn of their status until she is evacuated from University. Despite the uncertainty of her family's safety, she says there was nothing she could do about it. "If I concentrated on that, I would probably go crazy, so I just focused on the tasks at hand. I had so many people. We had three nurses who were so emotionally distraught that we had to take them out of duty. One of the nurses' daughter was a police officer and was involved in the explosion on the West Bank. She didn't know if she got hurt or was killed, so we took her out. Another nurse knew that one of her family members was in an attic and didn't know if they got out. They were concerned, so we just kept focusing on helping them, helping our patients."

The patient census is starting to swell, as several people make their way to the hospital once the storm passes. A few patients were discharged the Friday before Hurricane Katrina made landfall. There are 24 patients on the postpartum units. A pregnant woman arrives. There were no available beds. Gail says they get her a cot. Upstairs, there are 15 patients and double figures of babies between the two nurseries.

When employees venture outside on the ER ramp, the number of people who have not evacuated becomes evident. Recounts Gail, "We had people on their roofs, had people in the water. We had people who were trying to get to the hospital. Initially we were taking people in that could make it to the hospital. We were opening doors getting them in. It was quite a few."

An elderly woman is rescued by firefighters who are doing search and rescue. "She was an invalid, wheelchair bound," recalls Gail. "They found her in her bed and the fireman said the water was up to her nose. If she had been in there just a little while longer, she would have drowned in her bed. They brought her in. She was soaking wet. They found her wheelchair and brought it. Getting her in, getting her out of her wet clothes, getting a gown on her, getting her cleaned up, finding a bed for her, getting her in bed. It was pretty sad. She was alone in her house."

More people arrive in need of care. They are triaged on the hospital ER ramp. Once evaluated, they are given an identification bracelet. Rooms and resources soon reached capacity. On Tuesday night, the hospital locks its doors. However, still more patients come. This time they are deposited on the ER ramp by the military. "We are standing there looking out the window and we see them drive up—they put them on the ramp and leave!" says Gail. "We protested initially and said, 'Look, guys, we don't have beds, no stretchers, we are running out of food. We can't take anybody else. We don't have the resources.' It happened about three times; they'd just lay people on the ramp and leave and we had to go out and get them. I didn't believe that. But we went out and got them. We have to take care of them."

When she does try to rest, someone would call for her assistance. She stops eating but drinks water to stay hydrated. Many of the staff are concerned about leaving, about being rescued. It is important that she is visible and accessible to her nurses. "I couldn't just talk to the day people, I had to make sure that at night, when you go in talk to them, you just can't go in and say, 'Hey, how are you, got any questions?' and leave. You have to go in and sit down, talk to them, hear everybody, and let everybody vent and voice their concerns. And it wasn't just walking in and out and so, to be honest, that is what I spent 99% of my time doing—going around talking to people, making sure they were OK, making sure they got sleep, because they wouldn't sleep when their shift was over. They'd sit there, talk to the other staff, or walk around . . . forcing people to go sleep, go get a rest because you are going to have to take care of this baby and need to know you are rested enough to take care of this baby or take care of this mom."

She brings Incident Command Center briefings to her staff and assures all of them that they would be fine and would get out. "I was busy. I had a lot on my plate to worry about. To be honest, I wasn't really worried about me, and I'm an optimist. I wasn't just saying that I think we were going to get out; we were going to be OK. I felt that although we did get slammed with the storm, we were probably better prepared than we had been for any other storm, and I felt comfortable with the people who were here. . . . We were going to get what we needed in order to get out; it might not be as soon as we would like, but I felt comfortable we would make it and it would be OK."

On Thursday, September 1, administration is notified that helicopter evacuation is imminent. The hospital has no heliport. The roof is the only viable site for an air evacuation. Carrying the patients up the flights of stairs is physically taxing, but the wait is equally debilitating. Gail is told that rescue is coming. They wait for hours—no helicopters. One by one, the patients are carried back downstairs.

Friday morning, September 2, again, word comes that there would be an air evacuation. The patients are brought up to the roof. One patient requires 12 employees to move him. "You can't move a stretcher up, you can't move them in the stairwells," explains Gail. At every turn, a patient had to be lifted overhead because of the narrow stairwells.

No one knows if the roof has the capacity to bear the weight of a landing helicopter. It soon holds the weight of several helicopters that land as if in a choreographed dance. At one moment, when a full helicopter closes its doors and leaves, the patient who is next in line to board collapses, distraught that another helicopter might not be coming. Gail kept repeating, "Another one is coming, I promise."

With the final patient evacuated, it is time for the staff to go. As each floor is cleared, the staff are directed to get in line to leave. Gail's nurses are in the red group—the first group out. Their 29 babies have already made a successful evacuation. She tells her nurses they need to go. A few ask her to take their picture. They want a memento because they would not be there again. "I said, 'What are you saying? We are coming back,'" says Gail. "'We'll be back, and y'all will be complaining and taking too much break time.' They said, 'No, we don't think it's going to reopen.' I never believed that. I said, 'It will take a few months.'"

On Friday, in late afternoon, an exhausted but relieved Gail steps onto a boat, along with fellow administrators. Patients, family members, and employees are already evacuated. There is no one left at University Hospital. As the boat moves away from the hospital, Gail surveys the neighborhood. She is shocked by the sight of the water that has engulfed the city. The boat travels on Johnson Street and then turns on Tulane Avenue. A solider, armed with a machine gun, sits at the bow. Two military boats escort their boat as it makes its way toward City Hall near Loyola Avenue. It is the first time Gail feels fear.

They are brought to City Hall, where buses wait in line. Some of her colleagues take the bus that is going to the airport. Gail tells a fellow administrator that she does not have a good feeling about going to the airport. "I can see myself sitting in the airport 2 days waiting to get out because I knew they were bringing patients to the airport. Another bus was going somewhere they did not know. I said, 'I am not going to the airport. I will take my chances over here,'" she says.

She boards an air-conditioned bus. Bottles of chilled water and MREs are given to the passengers. The driver cannot tell her where they are going. She drills him: "Are we going to Baton Rouge? Shreveport? Anywhere in Louisiana?" He tells her Baton Rouge is closed for evacuees. She sits back as the bus leaves New Orleans. Her Palm Pilot is out. Her cell phone has no battery power. She begins her questioning anew.

The driver finally reports that their destination is Dallas. Gail asks if she can get off the bus before Dallas. "He said, 'I'll get in trouble. I can't let you off,'" she recalls. "I am sitting there saying most of my family is in Baton Rouge and Lafayette. So finally he calls the other bus driver, then he gets on the intercom and says, 'We're making a stop.' He asks how many people want to get out, and half of the bus says, 'Yeah, we want to get off. Thank you, thank you, thank you!'"

They are dropped off at a gas station and convenience store outside of Lafayette. It is Friday night. It has been 6 days since she last saw her husband. At the convenience store, she calls her family in Baton Rouge. Her oldest daughter answers the phone.

"I called the number where my daughters were going to be and I didn't know who else was there, and my oldest answered the phone," Gail says. "I say, 'Hi, this is Mommy.'"

On the other end, she hears her oldest start screaming. She can hear her youngest child crying. She tells them where she is. An hour later, she reunites with her family, who tell her she looks like a prisoner of war or refugee. It has been days since she had a shower. She has lost 16 pounds.

For 7 months, Gail and her family live in Baton Rouge while their home is repaired. She fills her days taking care of her children because their lives had been disrupted by the hurricane and its aftermath. Her other home, University Hospital, was closed. She thought she would be there for the remainder of her career, and now it is gone.

"All the people I had worked with for years, I had not been given the opportunity to tell them good-bye and good luck. You didn't get to leave on your own terms. I had not said good-bye to people I may never ever see again. . . . The hospital didn't open and they are not going to come back, so that was very disappointing."

There are work offers at other hospitals in the LSU Health System, but Gail declines. In March 2006, she receives a call. A sister hospital in Bogalusa is opening an obstetrics unit. They need someone to do the planning. Could she come? She says yes, but not on a full-time basis.

"I helped them from ground up," she states. "They did not have obstetrics and it was the first opening of the service in that city. Patients had to go to Covington, several miles away . . . so they had an opportunity to do very well if they put the unit together right."

The new job is over 100 miles one-way from her home. Three days a week, she commutes. She is asked to stay. Gail does not want to leave New Orleans. Another job offer comes. It is the one she wants. In December 2007, she returns to the shuttered University Hospital.

"It was very surreal coming back into the building after the storm and just looking around. Did we really leave things like that? Looked like we left in a hurry, things in disarray. Had suitcases in places you don't normally have them. Clothes taken out when someone had to pull what little they could to take with them when they left."

There also is a tremendous amount of mold in the basement and other places. Anyone entering the building is required to wear a mask for protection. She periodically goes to the closed and darkened Charity Hospital to retrieve items for use at University Hospital. Oftentimes she goes alone, armed with a flashlight. Returning to University Hospital is exciting and challenging. Gail works with contractors, vendors, and FEMA. The medical/surgical beds are opened first and obstetrics beds open next. All of Gail's managers eventually return to the hospital. Emergency services reopen in tents, then move into the Convention Center. They are relocated in the former Lord and Taylor store at the shopping center on Poydras, next to the Superdome.

At the time of this printing, University Hospital is not back to its prestorm strength. There are 20 beds open in the obstetrics unit. The 36-bed pediatrics unit remains closed. Gail says there was no choice but to reopen University Hospital.

"One bad storm in 25 years is not too bad and we made it through it. We did OK. Our patients made it through fine. It is important as a nurse, whether you are in a hospital because of a fire, hurricane, or earthquake, to take care of yourself so that you can take care of the people that you are responsible for. Keep your mind on what's going on and you can do OK and get out of it."

Mary Kelly

After Katrina, we didn't come back to answers because there was nobody who had ever experienced something like this. There was no one who wrote about how they handled certain situations. There is so much that comes out of this, but it is never enough because there is always information that you can use if you are ever put in a situation similar to it.

Mary Kelly, RN, MSN, MHA, began her nursing career in 1991 at Charity Hospital in New Orleans. She has worked in many areas and in various administrative capacities within the hospital, including medical/surgical, dialysis, infectious diseases, quality management, risk management, regulatory compliance, and patient care services. Mary is currently working as the clinical planning liaison at the Interim LSU Public Hospital, formerly University Hospital. Her responsibilities include working with an architectural firm to plan a new Academic Medical Center in downtown New Orleans. Mary serves as adjunct faculty for LSU's Career Alternative RN Education (CARE) program. She is also a trained parish nurse and leads the congregational wellness program at her church. Mary is interested in community outreach and improving health care access. Originally from New Orleans, Mary completed her initial nurse training at Charity School of Nursing and received her bachelor of science, master of science, and master in health administration degrees from the University of Phoenix.

On Friday, August 26, while the staff monitors the projected course of Hurricane Katrina, the hospital's code gray warning/activation phase begins. As many patients as possible are discharged. Mary, who is on the hospital's administrative team, reports to work on Sunday, August 28, at 5:30 A.M. She supervises the labor pool and cross-checks employees' assignments for the storm. Each unit distributes armbands to everyone at the hospital, including families of the staff. Family members automatically become part of the labor pool and will assist where needed. An area is assigned for children of employees.

The hospital plans a semi-lockdown by 10:00 A.M. because it is still in activation phase. Mary's mother, her sister, and her 17-year-old nephew come to the hospital. She situates them in a room in the adjacent medical office building and returns to hospital administration on the fourth floor. She sets up her work station at the secretary's desk near the CEO's office. The hospital census is approximately 200 patients.

Having worked other hurricanes, Mary anticipates nothing unusual with this one. "The first hurricane I reported for was Andrew," she says. "After each storm we would review what worked and what didn't. We would ask, 'Did we have enough supplies? Did our systems work?' We reviewed our plan and revised it after each event. Prior to Hurricane Katrina, we had started looking at contingency plans for Health Information Systems. Each time we had an event, we looked how to fine-tune things and make the plan better."

On Sunday, the Pharmacy Department is relocated to the medical library on the fourth floor. A large portion of supplies from the kitchen and central materials are moved from the basement. The computer management system is set up in the auditorium. Portable generators are stationed in key patient areas on different floors, including recovery and the ICU. Fuel for the portable generators is topped off. They are ready for use at a moment's notice.

Late Sunday, as the hurricane winds increase, everyone who is using the medical office building for sleeping quarters is told to move to the hospital because of concerns that the walkway that connects the two facilities may become compromised. Mary relocates her family.

On Tuesday morning, the water on the street rises continuously. The CEO calls a meeting with the administrative team. He informs them that there are breaks in the levees that protect the city from flooding. There is no time frame for evacuation. They communicate with Charity, their sister hospital, for additional planning. Hospital police and a few physicians take a small skiff to check out activity in the area.

"After the storm, it was like one of those horror stories and you are on the island. You look right down the street and know there is traffic in the distance. You are saying, 'We're dying and why can't we get out of here?'" Mary offers.

She says some nurses had the attitude that "we need to get through this." Others were overwhelmed from not knowing if their families were safe. "I saw this firsthand. Nurses and physicians would go to the CEO and tell him they needed to leave. You'd have to calm them down and tell them, 'Look what's out there. It's not safe for you to go.' Later, people told me what they remember is how I calmed them when they did not know what to expect. When I made my rounds I would say, let's get this done."

After the hospital loses electricity, the heat becomes oppressive. By Wednesday, August 31, Mary says, conditions worsen. The maintenance crew use sledgehammers to break windows. Mary says it only helps circulate foul-smelling air. When the CEO is directed by the military to evacuate the hospital to the Superdome, he refuses. Everyone will stay at the hospital, where they have resources.

As the days pass, a major challenge is to keep people calm and to assure them that there is enough water and food for everyone. When generators are refueled, nurses hand-bag the ventilator patients until they can reconnect to the power source.

"Supplies of food and water never ran out," Mary explains. "It just was the fact of not being able to leave, but needing to go.

"A lot of people wanted to feel OK," she continues. "They felt if you're OK, they are OK, but if you start to show any panic and you are supposed to be the lead, well then they are going to take your lead. I made rounds, up and down the stairs, checking on everyone. I'd ask how they were. I would tell them they're all doing a good job, keep up the good work. When I gave them information I would not give it to them too quickly because then, if it doesn't happen, they would tend not to trust you anymore. More than one time we were told we would be getting out, and then the news reports said we were gone. They don't even know we were still there."

The discovery of a working phone in the medical office building means contact with the outside. Mary sends her sister to wait in line with hospital employees and families to make one call. She reaches the family in St. Francisville, Louisiana, and assures them that they are OK. Her mother is relieved by the news that her other sister is safe and with family in Baton Rouge. Mary's mother joins a group that sings gospel songs for patients and employees on the fourth floor. The wait for evacuation draws into days. As she makes her rounds, Mary reassures employees that the administration team is in contact with their main hub at the central office in Baton Rouge. Help will come.

"You just had to keep saying we are going to get out. Can't give you a specific time when, but we are going to get out. People know that we are here. That's what they wanted to hear. If we started to panic, they would have, but as long as they came up and saw that we were talking, working, and reassuring them, they were OK."

The hospital evacuation plan calls for patient evacuation first. A color-coded system designates the various levels of patient acuity. A plastic bag that holds medications and notes from the patient's chart is pinned to each patient's hospital gown. The majority of patients leave by helicopter. On Tuesday, the babies in the third-floor nursery and NICU are evacuated via boat and helicopter. Next to leave are the ICU patients, followed by the renal patients. Some patients are transported by boat to Tulane for evacuation, but they return and are stationed in the first-floor ER and later evacuated via helicopter.

In 1991, when she began nursing at Charity Hospital, Mary recalls few "luxuries" and many opportunities to improvise. During the 6 days of confinement at University Hospital, she is grateful for the Charity experience and learning to use limited resources. Mary collects information from employees who need medications when the time comes to leave. Word travels quickly that physicians are writing prescriptions for staff. When they leave, no one knows their destination.

On Friday, September 2, Mary and her family leave. They are among the last group departing. Their boat slowly moves along Tulane Avenue. There is a clicking sound under the boat as the bottom skims across submerged cars. Past the corner of Galvez Street, a body floats in the water. The boat pulls up to a hotel where a military truck waits. Mary and the others press themselves inside the truck. Two soldiers, guns in hand, position themselves at the back of the truck. Their destination is the intersection of Causeway and Interstate 10.

"It looked like a postwar scene—like the survivors after a war where they are wounded," she relates. "They're dirty. Some of them are spaced out walking around. You see these movies with these people who are the last ones left on earth. Everything else is gone but now you are here. It was more like a camp setting where everybody had the same issues, but nobody had the solution. It was out of our control, and you just couldn't say, 'I need to go.' And the same highway that you traveled hundreds of times wouldn't get you to where you needed to be because they had blocked it off right there by Causeway. I had passed that way many times before. What was strange, my mother later could not remember which part of the bridge we were by—I had to show her. I told her, 'This is where we were, don't you remember?' She says, 'I am sorry, I don't. I only remember we came off a bridge.' I guess she blocked it out. The highway that took you west all those years, you are on it, but you can't go anywhere."

Still wearing their scrubs, Mary and the other nurses are motioned to a triage area. They are told they need to assist with eye irrigation of the men and women who gather under the overpass. Mary tries to explain that they have come from an evacuated hospital. It does not matter. She is just one of the thousands near the overpass. She takes the saline solution and IV tubing and starts working.

"Three of the nurses I was with just freaked out. Every time a helicopter landed, one person would tell you to do one thing, and then another directed you to the helicopter, telling you that you were not supposed to be there. I saw an elderly man who just dropped in front of me. I knew he was dead," she says. "I saw a lady whom I had known for years. She used to work at Dillard's department store, and she was just out of it. She didn't know who we were. She had been there for days."

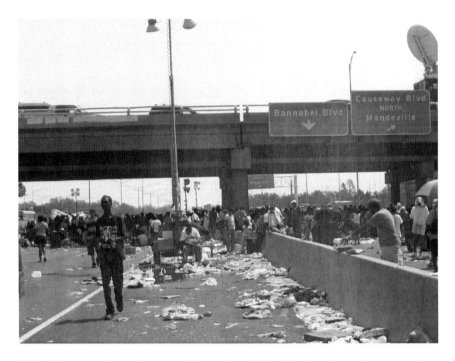

At the Interstate 10 and Causeway intersection in Metairie, Louisiana, thousands of evacuees were brought to a staging area for evacuation from New Orleans. Photo by Scarlett Welch-Nakajima

"I was tired, but I knew how my family relied on me," Mary continues. " I didn't want them to see me go off. It was bad enough that two of the nurses I was with I thought they were going to need medication. They are shouting at me to tell them we are not supposed to be there. Well, we were no longer at the hospital and had no choice. The military is saying, 'Don't move toward that helicopter.' Finally, the two nurses they jumped on a helicopter. That's how desperate they were."

After an hour and a half, Mary sees an employee of emergency medical services. He had worked at both Charity and University hospitals. He tells them where others are waiting to leave on a helicopter. They go there, but military personnel warn them that they cannot leave. Mary is resigned that they will stay, but the man returns later. He tells her to take her family and other hospital employees and walk to another area where the elderly are leaving for the airport. She does, and no one stops them.

"To this day, I have never seen the guy who told us to keep walking to get on the bus. Just because he recognized us he told us to keep walking," she says.

At Louis Armstrong International Airport, Mary's group catches up with other University Hospital personnel. Timing is fortuitous because minutes after she joins them, the line they are in is cut off. That evening, they board a C130 bound for a military base in San Antonio. At the base, they have to be processed, along with thousands of other evacuees. Tired, her last shower nearly a week ago, Mary tells a soldier that they are getting out of line. The man replies that he is responsible for her. Then her CEO appears and tells her that she can listen to the solider if she wants, but he is going to the Marriott. Mary and her family leave. While in San Antonio, Mary finally sees the news reports. There is news footage of boats launched from her neighborhood grocery. She knows that her home in Gentilly was claimed by the water. She reaches a hospital employee who worked in Environmental Services and is also a police officer. She asks if he can check on her mother's house. He sends back a report—the roses are blooming at her mother's home on North Lopez, not that far from where University Hospital is located. The house is fine.

From San Antonio, Mary and her family travel to Zachary, Louisiana, near Baton Rouge. They are there for 2 weeks, when her CEO calls to tell her that she has to report to work the next week at the Baton Rouge office. They have a hospital to reopen. In October, the administrative council returns to New Orleans to assess conditions. The hospital police are on-site, as is a National Guard unit. Administration works out of the Human Resources office in a nearby building across from Charity Hospital. They also work from a tent in a parking lot on South Johnson Street.

"I really don't know what kept me going, but I think a part of it was that I knew I wanted to be a part of the recovery and that we needed to come back to do something," she says. "There were patients who needed our services. From the family perspective, I had to be there for my mother because my father had died in 2004. At the hospital, I was the only person in regulatory compliance, so I knew I was needed to guide them on the regulations. It is a nursing thing. You need to do for everybody else."

At Mary's home in Gentilly, 13 feet of water has left its muddy mark. She finds her Charity School of Nursing pin and Great 100 Nurses pin. They are in a jewelry box inside a soggy shoe box. Other shoe boxes that floated during the flooding are embedded in a bedroom wall.

Mary moves in with her mother. She stays there for 3 years. During that time, she tries to rebuild her home, but it is eventually razed and the land sold. In December 2008, she moves into a new place near her old neighborhood.

Four years post–Hurricane Katrina, Mary acknowledges that some people may be weary about the subject. But she believes it is important to continue the discussion "because one day, if something happens to hospital personnel, they may be able to recall the experiences of nurses who went through this. After Hurricane Katrina, we didn't come back to answers because there was nobody who had ever experienced something like this. [Before] there was no one who wrote about how they handled certain situations. There is so much that comes out of this that it is never enough because there is always information that you can use if you are ever put in a similar situation. And now there are resolutions to some of the issues that nobody had before."

She has seen some of those resolutions with advanced communications systems and improved emergency preparedness plans. Today, hospital policy allows staff only to report during a hurricane evacuation—family members are not allowed. At University Hospital, building renovations have been made to improve flood protection.

"In 2008, with Hurricane Gustav, cable and electricity never went out, so that wasn't even a comparison to Hurricane Katrina," says Mary. "They made changes after Hurricane Katrina that made a difference in Hurricane Gustav."

For every hurricane season, she prepares. "As long as I get my family away to a safe place, I am OK. When I signed up for this, I knew what I signed up for. I agreed to report for a hurricane. I had how many years to decide I didn't want to do that?

"After Katrina, I had a new attitude, a new outlook on life. I can do anything. Just tell me what is needed. The hospital—we got it running. We had patients. We opened the psychiatric facility at DePaul and opened community clinics throughout the city. That is something we didn't have before."

She is on the hospital activation team. Mary's advice to anyone who may be faced with this situation is to focus on resources before the storm and safety during and afterward. At Interim LSU Public Hospital, she is now the planning liaison and works directly with the architectural firm, giving her clinical input on design, flow, and operations.

"I did not talk about Katrina until 4 years after the hurricane. I had friends from out of town who asked me, 'Did you cry?' I haven't cried yet. It is kind of like when you look at the full picture. I am here, I've got life, and my family is safe. When you look at all of that, the rest of it is junk."

Dan Kiff

I had worked during hurricanes, but never where I was lost by the fact that the hospital was surrounded by water and I have 36 ICU patients that needed to leave. So I was like, well, this is a new one. But I have to say as far as being the leader, I felt in my mind I had to show no emotion. I had to just stay positive and privately I was thinking, my God, I hope my family is OK. I hope my home is OK. I hope that this nightmare is going to end once I get out of here.

Dan Kiff, RN, MN, has been a registered nurse for 18 years. He received a diploma in nursing from Charity School of Nursing in May 1991, a BSN from the University of Alabama in December 1997, and a master of nursing degree from LSU Health Sciences Center in August 2005. Dan is presently employed at the Interim LSU Public Hospital (formally Charity Hospital) as the trauma program manager of the only Level 1 Trauma Center in the New Orleans area. His past job experiences have been in the medical ICU at Charity Hospital as a staff nurse, clinical coordinator, and RN manager.

During his 16 years at Charity Hospital, Dan Kiff had been through hurricanes before. He knows the drill. Plan for 3 days with a change of clothes and food. The storm would pass. Damage would be assessed. The relief team would take over and he could return home. But for this one called Katrina, intuitively, Dan prepares for the worst. He packs a suitcase with a week's supply of clothing, including a suit, just in case he would be job hunting if the hurricane destroyed the hospital. He leaves his personal papers locked in his truck, which he parks in the employee garage.

About three o'clock on the morning of Tuesday, August 30, the aftermath of Hurricane Katrina was not like the other storms. While he is deep in sleep, someone taps Dan's shoulder. Then he hears, "You need to wake up." Something had happened.

It is one of the charge nurses. Dan quickly gets up. The news is not good. There are breaks in the levees. The hospital is surrounded by water.

"I am thinking, my God, this is not good. How are we ever going to get out of this one? I knew that the water surrounded the city and everything had flooded out. I am thinking, 'How are we going to get the patients out?' I had an ICU with critically ill patients. In our ICU, we had a 21-year-old who was fighting for his life. I knew when the water got in and the power was out and he needed dialysis, this is going to get bad. And there were the two mothers who I allowed to stay in the family waiting room. I had to watch them every day. They would look me in the eyes and say, 'Are we going to get out of here? Are we ever going to get him out of here?' It was bad."

A generator is brought to his unit and they are able to power up the equipment to keep the patient alive. The hospital does not have a heliport. It has no boats. Power supply is limited. The staff can move the patients, but there are no ambulances. How do they get them out through water that is chest high?

By August 31, his fourth day at the hospital, Dan is furious. He tells the medical director that no one is coming to help. What is the plan?

"There were reports that we had been evacuated," says Dan. "So by Wednesday, I got angry. You know what? I don't care about public relations anymore; I don't care about not making a statement. If the nurses want to get on the telephone with CNN, do it!"

There are protocols to follow regarding media relations, but Dan says there were some very young nurses who could care less. The hospital is heavily damaged from the flooding, and most likely they will have no jobs to return to after they evacuate. Dan orders, "Give them a phone and let them say what they want to say."

"There was one nurse, about 22 years old. I had just hired her," he recalls. "She had been there about 6 weeks. She was devastated. I say, 'Listen, I have never been put in this situation. But I tell you what. I won't let anybody hurt you. We are going to fight together and get out of here. We are going to do that. The one thing I am not afraid of is our protection. We have police officers everywhere. We have an ex-marine on the unit with a gun.' I was not scared. If they get past this 6 foot 6 towering man, then I need to die. So I wasn't concerned and she wasn't scared for her safety. I think she was more afraid about her family. Again, everybody was worried about the unknown."

The nurses reach the news media. During a live interview, a nurse tells a reporter that she is at the hospital. They have patients and no one is coming to help. The news coverage prompts a response. A private helicopter service can assist. Dan's patients are in the surgical, medical, and neuro ICUs. He knows three patients must leave soon or they will not survive the hellish conditions at the hospital. One of the patients is a 14-year-old in the Neuro ICU.

"I had to get that patient out of there or he would die," relates Dan. "That night the owner of a private helicopter service called us saying they are willing to come and get them out of there. Whomever you think would not make it, we'll get them out."

The hospital's medical director makes a call, and arrangements are made for an ambulance for patient transfer once the helicopter reaches dry land. But the challenge is that the hospital has no heliport. Dan explains, "What happened was choreographed through several people. We actually commandeered a boat, and we were able to go across in the boat with the patient to Tulane Medical Center. They had a heliport. We brought the patient from the seventh floor, went down seven flights of steps, and brought him across the street. We got him to safety."

One patient out, Dan turns his attention to two other critically ill patients. He tells the medical director that if the heat is unbearable for the staff, imagine what the patients are feeling. They have got to get them out.

"I said, 'We have got to either call somebody else or ask these people if they can get someone else on the radio to help,'" Dan says. "And they did that. They got another helicopter. So, again, we did the boat trip and got them over there. That night was when I just said, 'We have to take matters in our own hands or we are never going to survive. We have got to get the patients out of here. I am able-bodied, but these people are not. We got a game plan.' And I said, 'Let's get the patients to Tulane so they will know that we're there, and maybe we can get the military involved.'"

When headquarters checks on their status, Dan tells the Baton Rouge office that he does not know how much longer they can last. Food and water are running out. They are low on fuel for the generators. His staff has concerns about their own families. Are they safe? Dan's parents had evacuated their home in Pass Christian on the Mississippi Gulf Coast. He knows the coast has been hit by the worst part of the storm and has brought storm surges in excess of 25 feet. His parents' home is probably wiped from its foundation.

"The whole time, I kept thinking to myself, 'God is not going to give me more than what I can handle. These poor patients are dying. Nothing is going to stop me.' And I kept telling my staff, 'I won't let anybody hurt you. Come to me, come find me. We are going to get out of this.'

"I internalized everything. If I don't think about them, then they're OK. That is one thing I don't have to worry about. I have to worry about what I need to do right now. I tell you what—it builds character. I think that maybe this was the wake-up call to me that this was the right profession. This is what I was put on this earth to do. I had started out as a business major. My parents said enough of this BS; you are not making good grades. We have an option for you. You are moving back to New Orleans and going to nursing school. My mother is a nurse. She said I know I won't have to worry about you. I didn't want to do it, but when I got into it, I realized this is for me."

Military help does come. Dan says a Tulane physician at the Superdome alerts them about ICU patients that needed to get to the heliport. The military brings their large deuce and half-trucks that can navigate the flooded streets.

"I had at least 17 patients vented. At this point, it is Thursday morning. Enough is enough! We have been put through hell; now it's burning hot, and we have to move all these patients out. We started moving the remaining patients out on the back of the trucks. I felt obligated to stay at Tulane because these are my patients. So, with another nurse and a respiratory therapist, we stayed to manage our patients. I didn't want Tulane to say, 'Some physician is using our area,' and then nobody is going to come and watch their patients," explains Dan.

From seven that morning, through the night, they work. Dan has lost contact with his staff at Charity. His last communication was when they started transferring patients out. He told them he would be at Tulane. They did not know he wasn't returning. He sends messages back to them. He does not know if they receive the messages.

"At first they thought I took off. Later, when it all came out what I was really doing, they were like, OK," he says. "I knew I had to have progress notes for each patient, and the staff was very smart. Each patient had a plastic bag with them. Inside the bag were progress notes, 5 days' worth of medicine, the patient's name, their card with all of their identification, list of any personal items they had because these patients could not communicate." As a Charity nurse now using the evacuation area for another hospital, Dan is acutely aware that his arrival with his patients is an unanticipated interruption for the Tulane staff. But he says they never made him feel he was on the opposing side.

"We kind of interrupted their evacuation," explains Dan. "We needed to have space for our patients, but we still allowed their patients to go first. These people gave me safety. And I was able to get my patients out. My job was to get them out to the best of my abilities by the grace and goodness of them.

"I think that we, as nurses, are trained to think about nothing else but the cause. It was nothing else but what was the task at hand. To not think of anything else," he adds.

The Charity patients lie on backboards placed below the top floor of the parking garage. Dan and his colleagues hand-bag their patients. Someone brings them a portable generator and a suction machine. The staging area by the heliport is crowded with employees and patients. Lights are taken down along the perimeter of the heliport because the chopper blades may knock them down. When it comes time to move their patients, they are lifted to a gurney. Then Dan and his colleagues run, pushing the gurney up a steep incline to reach the waiting helicopter. They crouch low as the helicopter blades turn. This is not the time to be clipped by a blade.

Two patients are placed inside a Black Hawk. Dan gets in. They are taken to the staging area by Lakeside Mall, at the intersection of Interstate 10 and Causeway. The patients are handed off to a medical team. Dan returns to Tulane's heliport. There are 30 more patients to evacuate. "I was exhausted. I don't know how I did it," shrugs Dan. "But this person did it. In my mind it was almost like somebody gave me the power to just keep going, don't stop. And the sad part again was I felt like an outsider because I was at Tulane Hospital and I was a Charity person. Some people were making comments. But I didn't want to take anything. I had my own water. Just save my patients. But they were very good to me to the point where they gave me a sandwich, and the other nurse who was with me I wanted to split the sandwich. They said, 'No, no, you can have the whole sandwich.' I didn't want to drink their water. They said, 'No, you're exhausted. You have been running up there all day.' I was sweating buckets."

After 12 hours of nonstop work, the last Charity patient is placed inside a helicopter. It is almost midnight. Dan surveys the rooftop area. No patients. He feels a weight lifted from him. Gunshots ring out close by. A sharpshooter is positioned by the heliport to protect the employees who remain. Dan says the soldier looks only 20 years old. "I looked him in the eyes and thought, 'My god, you are a child and you are here to protect us.' When he clicked his gun, I jerked in fear. He said, 'I am sorry. Do you need anything?' I told him, 'Please, don't click the gun again.' We offered him a bottle of water. He said he did not need it, he was self-contained."

A Tulane staffer comes up to Dan and his two colleagues. They are told, "It is very dangerous out there; there is no way to get you back to Charity tonight."

"He said, 'You should not go. It is not a good idea,'" relates Dan. "'You can stay with us, but if you step foot off this property, if something happens, you can't come back. We will protect you now, but once you leave the property you are on your own.'

"I felt I did my job. All the patients were gone. It was cool on the roof. There was a guy in a hotel next door from where we were in the Saratoga Garage. This man watched us taking the patients out. He said it is amazing what we have done. From a hotel window, he threw pillows to us. I thought that was wonderful.

"That night I slept. I remember hearing a few explosions and thought, man, what is on for tomorrow? No more helicopters came. It was dark, too dangerous to fly. We couldn't go anymore. We all slept. Friday morning, I told myself I made it through the night. My job was done. I got the patients to safety."

Dan wonders what is happening at Charity Hospital. Again, he is given the offer to leave with the Tulane employees. The choice is a difficult one. What about his staff? The military helicopters are gone. No one wants to go to Charity Hospital. The only option is to walk to Charity in the water.

"I went to our medical director. He is like my father, my family. I told him, 'They are giving me the option to leave.' I said, 'I feel terrible about this. I am exhausted. I can't go anymore. I am not walking in water. They tell me it is very dangerous out there.' People were breaking into places. I did not feel comfortable. We had made it this far; I don't want to get shot. I made the decision, I did my job, now I am going to go.

"A physician from Tulane said you have done all that you can do. In your mind, if you feel you want to walk those waters into a hostile environment, you do that, but I think you've done enough. There comes a time the leader has to take care of the leader. I told him, 'But I am the leader.' He replied, 'Yes, but your staff is going to be taken care of. Everybody now knows what is down here. They are going to get them out.'"

Dan decides to leave with the Tulane employees. "They will take me to safety," he offers. "Heaven had opened up at that time. To me, life was going to get better immediately. It was the hardest decision I ever made, but when he told me it is time for the leader to take care of the leader, I knew it was time to leave."

Dan and the others are flown to Louis Armstrong International Airport. From there, they are taken by chartered buses to a hospital in Lafayette, Louisiana. Because of his exposure to contaminated flood waters he goes through the decontamination process, and is given clothing, shoes, food, and a place to sleep. An ER resident tells him her father is coming from Dallas to get her and her colleagues. Dan needs to go with them to Dallas. He doesn't have to worry about the details. The physician tells Dan, "You are my people, and we are going to take care of you."

On Sunday, he reaches his parents. Their home is gone, but they can rebuild. He gets a call from one of his staff members.

"At the same time I was leaving Tulane, my staff was leaving," relates Dan. "I did not know that until Sunday morning when one of my staff got me and said, 'Dan, they all got out. They know what happened. They were upset with you, but they know that you didn't leave them.'"

Of the 36 ICU patients they had evacuated, Dan says 3 died. They lost two on the heliport while waiting to evacuate. A month after Katrina, Dan returns to New Orleans and Charity Hospital. With him is a crew from the television news program *20/20*. They go to his office. Two weeks before the hurricane, Dan had graduated with his master's degree in nursing. He says it is weird seeing his papers and personal effects in the office untouched. He thinks, "This was my life. It is over, gone."

Soon after his return to the city, the staff has a reunion. They debrief one another. They talk about their future. "There are people I am going to be friends with for the rest of my life because of what I had to share with them. Like the doctor whose dad drove from Dallas to get us. I see her and ask, 'How's your dad? I will never forget what he did for me.' We had a great unit, and through no fault of mine, I had good people who surrounded me."

In February 2006, Dan returns to work as trauma program manager. The hospital has to reinstate its Level 1 Trauma Center designation and Dan brings to the job his experience in the verification and accreditation process. In November 2008, the hospital is back to Level 1 status. Only five of his former staff members return. It is slow the first weeks after reopening, but soon, they are at capacity.

For Dan, his return to work is a homecoming to a place where he has spent his entire adult life—from nursing school to his first job. He is hopeful that others will benefit from those who dealt firsthand with Katrina.

"With this unstable weather that we have everywhere, others need to learn from our mistakes," he says. "We made mistakes, but we learned from them. The biggest thing they need to learn is that communication is the key to everything. If you lose communication with the outside world, you suffer. Why is it that nobody came? I would go to meetings thinking, 'We are here, why don't they come?' You have patients that are your priority. That's why it takes a very special person to do this job. You had better have the character to do this. If you don't, then you would have just left and abandoned them. I was there being paid for a job to take care of patients. Now, I may have not been the caregiver to them, but it is funny how your skills never leave you. I was exhausted, and I am thinking, 'I am as good as the best of them.' It is still in my head. The young nurses were looking at me as I rolled with the punches. Nothing bothered me. You have got to do it and move! Don't cry about it; you don't have time. I now know how to fuel a generator. In the real world, it was life's lessons learned. I was able to do things that I thought I would not be able to do."

Those 6 days at Charity Hospital changed Dan. It gave him a new perspective. "I think it was the first time I realized this was probably the profession I needed to be in. Once it all happened and it broke, I was probably one of the senior leadership people in the hospital taking care of what I didn't know how to take care of. I mean, I had worked during hurricanes, but never where I was lost by the fact that the hospital was surrounded by water and I have 36 ICU patients that needed to leave. So I was like, well, this is a new one. But I have to say, as far as being the leader, I felt in my mind I had to show no emotion. I had to just stay positive, and privately I was thinking, 'My God, I hope my family is OK. I hope my home is OK. I hope that this nightmare is going to end once I get out of here.' But I never talked about that with others. I never said, 'Oh, my God, this is horrible,' because I didn't want them to be upset. I just wanted to keep my mind on our task at hand. Get these people to safety so I could go home. My first priority. I say it changed me because it made me realize that my profession had changed me as a person. The people that I was taking care of, they were my first priority at that time. Although I have a family, the task at hand is what I needed to do. My whole thought process was getting patients to safety."

3 Lindy Boggs Medical Center

Lindy Boggs Medical Center traces its roots to Dublin, Ireland, and Catherine McAuley, who was born there in September 1778 to a prosperous Roman Catholic family. Her father, James McAuley, died when she was 5 years old. Even at that early age, he had impressed on her his compassion for the poor. When she was orphaned in 1798, Catherine lived with relatives. Not all of them were Roman Catholic, nor did they approve of her pious way of life.

In 1803, she accepted an invitation from William and Catherine Callaghan to live in their home, where she would be a companion for Mrs. Callaghan. When William Callaghan died in 1822, he had no children. He bequeathed his estate to the young Catherine. She used her inheritance to respond to the needs of the sick and the poor and leased a building to open a home for religious, educational, and social services for women and children. The House of Mercy welcomed its first residents on September 24, 1827, the feast day for Our Lady of Mercy. On December 12, 1831, Catherine founded the Community of the Sisters of Mercy (Sisters of Mercy of the Americas, 2006a).

The order came to the United States in 1843 and, in 1869, opened a school for children and also a local clinic in New Orleans. In 1924, Mrs. Leonce Sonait donated her estate on Annunciation Street to the

Sisters of Mercy, where the hospital was originally located (Sisters of Mercy of the Americas, 2006b).

Mercy Hospital moved to the corner of Jefferson Davis Parkway and Bienville Street in 1953. Over the next decades, it added a convent and expanded the hospital to include an adjacent medical office building.

In 1994, Mercy Hospital merged with Southern Baptist Hospital to become Mercy + Baptist Medical Center. The merger created the largest private hospital in the metropolitan area, with 726 beds and a dual-campus geographic advantage. The management of the facilities also merged to become Christian Health Ministries, and the two medical staffs became one.

While the merger helped to strengthen the position of the institution financially, the leadership of Christian Health Ministries began to see the evolution of large health care systems, or partnerships, emerging in the market. These partnerships were combining multiple hospitals and using their leverage to negotiate managed care contracts. Additionally, pressures to reduce both health care costs and charges also became a concern among hospital leadership.

By 1995, it was decided that Mercy + Baptist could not stand alone in the New Orleans market. It needed a partner that could position the medical center at the center of a growing network. After reviewing three options, including a partnership with a group of New Orleans–area nonprofit hospitals, or acquisition by one of two for-profit hospital chains that included orNda and Tenet Healthcare Corporation, Christian Health Ministries decided to sell the facility to Tenet Healthcare Corporation; a name change was one of the conditions of the sale. In August 1996, Mercy Hospital became part of Memorial Medical Center Baptist and Mercy campuses.

In 2003, the dual-campus medical center separated. The Mercy campus was renamed Lindy Boggs Medical Center, in honor of the former Louisiana congresswoman who also served as U.S. ambassador to the Vatican from 1997 to 2001.

The 187-bed hospital sustained significant damage from flooding caused by Hurricane Katrina. In May 2007, Tenet announced it sold the hospital to Victory Real Estate of Columbus, Georgia. The new owner planned to develop the land for mixed-use retail. It was later reported that the sale of Lindy Boggs Medical Center was part of an agreement between the former owner and Ochsner Health System, which had purchased three other hospitals owned by Tenet. A local newspaper reported that the sales contract contained a resolution that spelled out the building's future: "Upon acquisition of the Property, the Company will demolish Lindy Boggs Medical Center and re-development [*sic*] the Property."

Tenet had agreed with Ochsner to prevent whoever bought Lindy Boggs from using the site for certain health care purposes for 3 years after the sale, according to Tenet. The property could be sold for "sub-acute" care purposes, such as the development of a clinic, but the creation of a private full-service hospital or other acute-care building was off limits unless Ochsner reviewed and approved the plans (DeGregorio, 2007).

As of summer 2009, Lindy Boggs Medical Center remains shuttered.

Four nurses recount what they experienced during their last days at Lindy Boggs Medical Center before the permanent closure of a place where they had worked for so many years.

Roslyn Pruitt

I am up on the roof trying to figure out what the hell is going on. I am looking and everything is black. In a giant city where there is noise all the time. The blackness. Except for the gunshots and the screaming and more gunshots and more screaming. I am like, what the hell! Oh my god, it is Armageddon. It is close, very close.

Roslyn Pruitt, RN, entered health care in 1975 as a nurse assistant and became an emergency medical technician in 1976. She has worked in emergency medical services (EMS) and hospital environments and has been a health facilities surveyor for Centers for Medicare and Medicaid Services in the states of California and Louisiana. She is married, has four grown children, and lives in New Orleans, Louisiana. She is currently working as the director of clinical quality improvement for a medical center in Slidell, Louisiana.

Roslyn Pruitt's career track in nursing began with the EMS in the 1970s. She was among the first emergency medical technician (EMT) paramedic class in Southern California, where she took her first training in 1975. For several years, she worked as a paramedic in California, where paramedics work both in the field and, if they are part of an air medical transport team, in the emergency room (ER). That combination gives a "huge perspective," says Roslyn.

California is where the Incident Command System (ICS) developed. Roslyn took the first training for ICS in the 1980s. In 1992, she became a mobile intensive care nurse at a hospital in Chico, California, but still maintained her certification in EMT. Later, she worked for the federal government as a surveyor of nursing homes, hospitals, and ambulatory services. An offer to be a hospital compliance officer brought her to New Orleans, and in 2003, she joined the staff at Lindy Boggs Medical Center.

"It is an interesting set of experiences that gave me a very unique perspective of disasters. I have been in several disasters out in California. I have been on the field end of it. I have been on the government and hospital end of it. I have been on every end of it. I know how things work and how likely [they are] to fall out."

On Saturday night, August 27, Roslyn had vacation plans on her mind when she saw a weather update on Hurricane Katrina. The storm's massive size alarmed her. "I felt there is something bad that is going to happen and I am not a worrier," she says. "It is not in my nature. I am really good in a huge disaster. I am calm, but that's my niche. . . . That's why I am OK in the field and OK in the ER. I will fall apart afterwards—during it I am just fine."

By Sunday morning, she has packed her clothes for work. It is 6:00 A.M. when she tells her husband, Charles, good-bye, leaves their home on the West Bank, and heads for Lindy Boggs Medical Center in the Mid-City area of New Orleans. Charles will not be far behind her, but he is headed to the sister hospital of Memorial Medical Center, where he is director of environmental services. The two hospitals are less than 5 miles from each other.

Lindy Boggs Medical Center seems to be near a full patient census despite the early discharges and surgery cancellations that had begun Friday in preparation for the storm. Roslyn starts making rounds on each floor. Conversation with the charge nurses focuses on shift change, which can be critical if a hospital has no immediate relief after a storm makes landfall. There are 800 people in the hospital, including 120 patients. A total of six physicians have come to the hospital to work the storm. Roslyn says others doctors had promised to come but were no-shows.

A hospice facility leases the hospital's fourth floor and works independently, with its own staff. Seven of the hospice patients are ventilator-dependent. The hospice patients are terminally ill and in frail condition.

Roslyn hears there are concerns about the number of staff reporting to work at the hospice. The hospital includes the hospice patients in the total patient census of the hospital. The hospice administrator and other hospice employees coordinate communications with the Lindy Boggs staff.

On another floor was a long-term acute-care hospital with many ventilator-dependent patients, which was operated independently from Lindy Boggs Medical Center. The hospital includes them in the total patient census, as well.

It is early afternoon, and Roslyn raises her concerns about the ventilator-dependent patients with the hospital chief nursing officer. If the hospital loses power, who will hand-bag those patients? Can they get the very sick ones out of the hospital before the storm comes?

"Well, she did. She tried very hard to get them out of there. And no one would help us. EMS wouldn't help, med transport wouldn't help. Nobody would help," recounts Roslyn.

A call is made to the Emergency Operations Center (EOC) of Orleans Parish. The EOC tells them they are on their own and to stay in place. "That was devastating. It was an eye-opener for me at that point. If I wasn't alarmed before, I was even more alarmed, because the reality is there is a whole group of people who have never gone through this before—who don't really understand [what it] means—and the Emergency Operations Center can't help us. We lose power, and have all of these people, so I was fairly alarmed, more so at that point."

A few more patients arrive at the hospital. The police bring an elderly woman who had decided to stay at her home and ride out the storm. Roslyn tries to make sense of the situation. She asks the police if they can take the woman to a safer place. They ignore her request and leave their passenger at the hospital. The ER staff report receiving more patients from EMS and a community shelter.

"What did they think was going to happen when they got there?" she asks. "There is very poor communication between the hospitals and EMS. Some of the nurses in this state need to get their act together, and start meshing and working with, and develop some kind of fieldwork for nurses here, and talking to them about that as they do in other states. We need mobile intensive care nurses very badly. Here you are 20 years behind. It is unbelievable.

"They have to get with EMS. They need to know what is going on out in the field. They need to have a hand in, and understanding of, and have control over how things get to their ER because we are going to end up in the same place where we are at now, dropping those 20 patients off. Nurses have to step up and say, 'You know, we need some control over this.'"

By Sunday afternoon, hospital administrators close the ER as a measure to prevent future compromise of hospital resources. Anticipating power loss, they set up a cascade system with H tanks and also use intermittent positive pressure breathing devices for the patients who are ventilator-dependent. The machinery can help give the staff a break from hand-bagging the patient.

As she makes her second round through the hospital, Roslyn encounters family members. She strongly encourages them to leave. "I told them the hospital was not really a good place to be. 'If you can get out of town, this is the time to do it, leave. Do not be here.' Although the hospital is rated for 130 [winds], 'we cannot provide food, we cannot provide water. You need to go buy something now if you want to stay. We are not going to provide anything for you or your animals; I *don't* know where you are going to sleep. We don't have accommodations. We are not a hotel.'"

Despite her warnings, they choose to stay. She reflects on the numerous EOC meetings she had attended in the preceding months. The hospital had one boat—the Mercy boat. Roslyn relates that in California, residents can expect an earthquake at a moment's notice. At the meetings, she had stressed the need to be ready at any time.

On Sunday afternoon, the administration's hospital emergency plans are reviewed again. Threat of flooding is a major concern. The hospital basement houses the morgue, housekeeping, pharmacy, and the kitchen. Housekeeping supplies, pharmacy, and its refrigerator are moved upstairs. The kitchen supplies and food are relocated to the fourth floor, where the convent kitchen is located. The convent also has rooms for a handful of nuns in the Sisters of Mercy order. One nun has brought to the hospital her elderly mother, who has a feeding tube. Roslyn instructs the nun how to use it.

On Sunday night, the feeder bands of the storm arrive. Roslyn describes the winds "howling like a banshee." The windows in an elevator shatter. Debris of shingles and rocks becomes missiles in the high winds. Patients are moved from their rooms to the protected hallways when the windows begin to blow out from the debris hitting them.

In the boardroom on the first floor, hospital administrators review the day's events and monitor the storm's progress. There is some street flooding. A barrier on the loading dock is raised to prevent water from entering the basement. The water ebbs, but slowly inches over the sidewalk. In the early hours of Monday morning, the brunt of the storm has arrived. Roslyn steps outside under a protected entrance to watch.

"People were still in denial about what was reality at that point. They are used to seeing the flood. It dropped a little bit, but then it started coming up again . . . the worst part was hitting very early Monday morning. I went outside where it is protected. The trees are coming down, signs, wind was sideways. . . . I am the kind of person who needs to know what my surroundings are, what I have available if I need it. I am looking around thinking, 'Where is bottled water around here? . . . wait a minute, we are not going to have flushing toilets.'"

The storm has taken out the power and the generators are operating. The switching panels for the generators are housed in the basement, which is watched continuously for any signs of water seepage. The Incident Command Center is set up on the first floor. A small black-and-white battery-operated TV is monitored for news updates on the city's condition. Phone lines are not working. Overhead paging is relying on generator power. The final page bellows through the hospital: "All administrative teams *stat* to the basement."

When they reach the basement, Roslyn and her colleagues see water cascading over the barricade like a waterfall. Questions fly. How many minutes do we need before it hits the switching panels? How long do we have on emergency power?

"It's all bad. It's downhill from there," says Roslyn. "Monday night was scary. We had no power. Eight hundred people. The water was so high you had to swim to get to the hospital. There is gunfire. More gunfire. Screaming. More screaming. I am up on the roof trying to figure out what the hell is going on. I am looking, and everything is black. In a giant city where there is noise all the time. The blackness. Except for the gunshots and the screaming and more gunshots and more screaming. I am like, 'What the hell! Oh my god, it is Armageddon. It is close, very close.'"

The group returns to the boardroom. Roslyn turns to the CEO. "You understand that we're the victims now," she tells him and the others. Incident Command is moved to the second floor, where natural light filters into a small training classroom. Roslyn is the incident commander. A cardiologist and vice chief of the medical staff, is designated emergency chief of staff. Internal resources are reassessed. Volunteer help is recruited among family members and other guests. A set of radios is used between security and engineering. A runner system is set up to relay communications throughout the hospital. Flashlights light the way along the darkened hallways and stairwells and illuminate patient care areas. Roslyn uses a penlight to make her way to each floor as she makes her rounds.

The hospital is an island, isolated from any word of rescue. Inside, the temperature is over 100°. On Tuesday, at 2:00 A.M., one of the kitchen staff is in the fourth-floor convent dining area. He hears the sound of a helicopter. It sounds near, very near. Suddenly, a white light shines through the wall of windows that face South Jefferson Davis Parkway. The employee bolts from the room and races down the stairs to the Incident Command Center. He is shouting, "Roslyn, Roslyn, they are here!" Roslyn and others follow him back to the fourth floor. She waves her arms toward the light.

"I yelled, 'Help, help!' Do you think they did anything? Do you think they recognized us? Nothing," she says.

The helicopter leaves. Back in the boardroom, the administrative team tries to piece together the sketchy information they are receiving. There is talk about an explosion. Rumors are rampant but cannot be denied or confirmed. The hospital is in a communications vacuum. Some employees receive text messages. There is a break in the levees.

"It wasn't anything that said, 'Well, the levees broke; you need to get the hell out of there.' There was nothing like that," says Roslyn.

The runners and doctors canvass the floors, alerting staff and visitors to stop drinking the tap water because of likely contamination. They also advise them about infection control. Some people who had been in the floodwater on Monday night are showing signs of infection 8 hours later, with redness and visible streaks around the sites that had been exposed to the water.

"We were limited on antibiotics. If you can imagine, you have 800 people and everything is contaminated by then. We made sure everybody had hand gel and anybody who had contact understood they had to report nausea, vomiting, diarrhea, or fever immediately so that we could isolate them. We had people rotating through to make sure the precautions were followed because we had no overhead, no phones, no pagers, anything.

"We preached and we made round three times a day—wash your hands, wash your hands. Of course, the other problem was trying to get people to not turn on the water and/or try to flush the toilets. The minute that happens, we are going to get sewage backed up. So we put bags in every toilet to bag the waste."

On Monday, Roslyn decides to stop eating. She would sustain her energy with a few bites from an energy bar and with bottled water and vitamin water. In efforts to extend the food supply, meals are cut down to two a day. The nine dialysis patients are immediately placed on an emergency diet of limited fluids and food. The measures work to buy extra time for them.

On Tuesday, one of the residents tells Roslyn that they could use candles as a light source. She replies, "No, not a chance can you use these. We are in a building surrounded by water. We have 800 people and 150 of them need help. Really, you want to use a match and fire? Really?" She orders him to hand over his lighter and every match he has. She confiscates every candle.

The supply of antibiotics is running low. Someone suggests availing the supply at a nearby pharmacy. Roslyn is not ready to give her blessing. However, there are physician offices in the medical office building connected to the hospital. A group of employees make their way through 5 feet of water to secure medications from the offices. They bring them to the pharmacist.

By Tuesday, August 30, there are still no communications from outside. Then they hear the helicopters. One block away at the American Can Company condos, helicopters are landing to pick up people who have gathered on a dry grassy path by the post office.

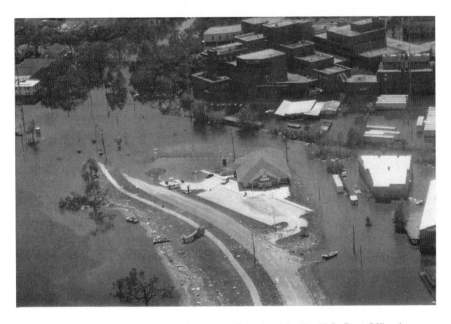

An aerial photograph shows the small patch of dry land by the U.S. Post Office in Mid-City New Orleans. Behind the post office is the flooded campus of Lindy Boggs Medical Center. Photo by Eric Yancovich.

"I said, 'Why are they picking people up from the Can Company when we have patients here that are going to die if they don't pick them up! I don't understand that!'" says Roslyn.

With no word of rescue coming, Incident Command decides to find boats from the neighborhood. The radiology director and others set out to acquire additional boats. If they can bring their patients to the post office, maybe more helicopters would come. By the end of the day, they have successfully brought the women, children, and some staff to the pickup area.

On Wednesday, early afternoon, around 1:00 P.M., members of the Shreveport Fire Department, with a fire unit from Tennessee, maneuver their boats to the hospital. The firefighters are incredulous to discover the patients and staff inside.

"They asked, 'Are you a hospital?'" relates Roslyn. "I said, 'You have got to be kidding me, right? Yes, we are a hospital.'"

One of the first questions they ask her is how many patients with do not resuscitate (DNR) orders they have. Roslyn replies, "You know what, here's the thing. I am a DNR. Are you really not going to save me? Really? Do you understand? That means you do everything for me until I code, and then you can tell me to shove off. Until then, what difference does it make? But that's what they asked. In their minds, a DNR is a comfort-care patient; that's not what it is and we need to get our language straight first of all and get over that."

The firefighters explain to the administrative team that this is a mass casualty incident. They will follow field triage for the hospital's evacuation. Those who can walk on their own or with assistance will leave first. Some of the hospital nursing staff are unfamiliar with field triage. They understand emergency medicine. You work to save the most critically ill.

Recalls Roslyn, "Some people asked me why they were doing it this way? I said, 'Do you understand we are the victim. This is field triage. This is the reality of field triage. You have to understand what field triage is. This is how it's going to be.'"

The firefighters review the hospital census on each floor. Patients are assigned to three groups: A, for ambulatory patients who can walk on their own; B, for those patients who can sit up or are in wheelchairs; and C, for those patients who are the most critically ill and at risk of dying during an evacuation. Many on the hospital staff are visibly upset with the plan. This is disaster medicine. The evacuation begins, and the patients are boarded on boats that wait by the back loading dock. At first, each person is given a tag, but when they run out of tags, a marker is used to write assigned letters on the person's forehead.

Each patient is given a triage tag. A summary of their medical chart is placed by them. Around their neck hangs a small plastic pouch with a 3-day supply of medication and their list of medications and how they should be given. "Enough information so that whoever got them could take care of them right there," Roslyn explains. "If they had a glass of water they could take care of them right there. That was the point.

"The staff was phenomenal. They did really step up in a huge way. They got people lined up in the back, the boat just came right up, they got on and then they went around to the post office about a quarter mile away. So we lined up the boats, lined up the patients, walked them down, put them in—take them around, take them out. It was reported back to me, 'Why are these patients here?' 'Well, there is a hospital there.' 'Where is there a hospital?' 'See that building right there?' I am thinking, 'Holy cow!'"

Darkness is descending. It is nearly 7:00 P.M. Nearly 400 people, including most of the 120 patients, have been evacuated. One of the lead firemen finds Roslyn. She has a vivid memory of how large his eyes were as he tells her they have been ordered to leave and stop the evacuation. There are reports of gunfire. The city is not safe. They were ready to evacuate everyone, but now the orders are to leave.

"I said, 'But not all the patients are out.' He says, 'I know. We are being ordered out.' I said, 'What?' 'We are being ordered out. We are being shot at. They have ordered us to leave.' I said, 'You are going to leave us here to be shot at?' And he said, 'Yeah.' 'You are leaving?' 'Yes.' 'Are you coming back?' 'No.' 'You are not coming back.' 'No, we are not coming back.' 'You know there are still patients here, right? And you are not coming back.' 'No.' 'Please, please come back. Because we need help getting the rest of the patients out.'"

She pauses. "So he leaves. They leave. I have to tell Incident Command. That was hard. Wednesday night, they left without us. Some of our security and staff had left earlier during evacuation to accompany patients. The fire department left and they said they weren't coming back. And all I know is we still have many patients and no help on the way."

News that the evacuation had halted stun those who were left. There are 30 patients to care for and 80 employees and family members at the marooned hospital. It is an otherwise quiet night, until Roslyn is notified that a friend of one of the nurses has thrown a rock through one of the windows in the intensive care unit.

"He decided that he sees people walking across the roof and he wants to get to another part of the hospital so he throws a rock so he can walk through. I told security to go get him. Nobody is going to risk the staff or patients. I don't care who they are. I don't care who they're with."

Security brings the man to Incident Command in handcuffs. Roslyn tells him, "'Here is the problem. We have no extra staff to watch this guy doing things that are endangering everybody here. We have people out there with guns trying to get in, so here's what we are going to do. You, sir, need to leave the premises. I don't care how you get out of here. Security, you escort him out the door and you put him into the water if you need to, but he's not going to endanger our staff. He's not.' So I did make that decision. I'm OK with it."

On Wednesday night, Roslyn feels the gravity of the situation. "Wednesday was bad," she says. "That was the first time I kind of cracked a little when they left us. Damn. *They left us!* They left us because it was too dangerous for them! What do they think it is for us? . . . We decided we were just going to move them out on Thursday ourselves."

Early Thursday morning, the hospital Incident Command regroups. They are resolved that everyone in the hospital will leave that day. They know the helicopters will be flying at daybreak. "Shame on them if they avoid us being out there, waving at them with white sheets and patients down here. Shame on them if they do that," says Roslyn.

They load the boats and ferry patients, family members, and staff to the grassy area by the post office. Only five patients who were too critical and frail to move remained. They would wait for medevac helicopters for these patients. A physician and a nurse stay at the hospital with the patients, who have been moved down to the first floor. The next morning, the remaining patients, physician, and nurse would be taken away from the hospital.

It is almost dark when Roslyn climbs into the boat. On the grassy patch by the post office, the last of the evacuees huddle together. And then helicopters start coming. It is windy. They are Black Hawk helicopters. "Security was fabulous. I told them, 'I don't think you understand how dangerous this is—hot on-load, hot off-load; very dangerous. Just duck and don't stand up. Duck!'"

Each helicopter can take about 20 people. It has been over 8 hours since they started the evacuation, and it is now getting dark. They all know that the helicopters stop flying at nightfall. Roslyn climbs aboard one of the last helicopters. As they leave, none of them knows they are about to go to another hellish place. Some of them are dropped off at the Louis Armstrong International Airport. Others go to the Convention Center. Roslyn is left at the intersection of Interstate 10 and Causeway in Metairie. She describes it as a scene from the movie *Apocalypse Now*. Helicopters hover, waiting to land and quickly unload their goods. Sometimes, two land at the same time. As soon as they leave, another helicopter arrives to deposit its human cargo. The evacuees from Lindy Boggs Medical Center are now among thousands of people who have been removed from the flooded area. Roslyn asks someone about a Red Cross station. She is told that Red Cross personnel had left because it was too dangerous.

"Here we are, coming in our scrubs to a place where thousands of people were, looking like medical help, and we were disasters ourselves. And people with wheelchairs started wheeling up to us. That's when I said to myself, 'We are screwed. There is no protection out here. Nothing out here.' There was no cover. There was no water. There was no food. We are dead dog-tired. There was no one in charge. There was no medical assistance. There was nothing except thousands of people. And about a hundred buses. A whole bunch of buses with drivers in each bus, standing there waiting. I don't know what the hell they were waiting for."

By now, she has joined with her colleagues who arrived ahead of her group. They centralize everyone in the middle of the interstate grassy strip. They need to leave. Some of them approach one of the buses. It is vacant. They ask the driver how much money it will take for him to take them out of there. Cash is collected for their passage and they board the bus. They arrive at a shelter in Baton Rouge. It has been 5 days since Roslyn last spoke with her husband. She wonders if he is OK. A colleague's son meets them at the shelter and takes some of them to Alexandria, Louisiana. Her colleague loans Roslyn cash. She had left the hospital without her credit card and money. That night, she takes four showers. She falls asleep. It is not restful. She dreams of boats and helicopters and the sounds from them that she heard every night while at the hospital. The intensity of her nightmares will gradually wane over time.

On Friday morning, she reaches her mother. No one has information about Charles. She tells her mother she is fine. "That's what you tell everybody, even if you're not," she says. Roslyn is worried sick about her husband.

In a happenstance way, she is able to find Charles. Someone text-messaged an employee at Memorial Medical Center, who was able to reach the sister hospital in Slidell at NorthShore Regional Medical Center. Some people in Roslyn's group are returning to Slidell and will try to find him. When they arrive at the hospital, Charles is on a bus waiting to leave for Dallas. "He heard someone walking by calling, 'Charles Pruitt, Charles Pruitt.' He said, 'Wait, I have to get off the bus,' and he found them that way. And I got a text message around Friday 2:00 A.M. It was nice to see him. I was toast. I was tired."

"He told me about all of the people he helped to carry up the stairs. . . . He had left his phone, his wallet, his computer, his clothes . . . everything, in his basement office (which was underwater). He had nothing with him. He decided he was going to go out on the last helicopter. He got to NorthShore."

The two of them have a week to recoup before they return to work. Charles is assigned to Beaumont, Texas. Roslyn stays in Dallas for a week of training and returns to their home.

Her mother, also a nurse, asks her if she would be part of the activation team for another hurricane. Roslyn replies yes. "Part of my job is to be here with people who need me. I am unique, so the experience qualifies me to be here. I am sorry, but why would I leave? This is my community. These are people that I care about. Nobody should just step down like that. I care about the patients. I care about the people who work there. Why wouldn't I?" she offers.

She remains concerned about a false sense of security people may have about future disasters, even those who experienced firsthand the aftermath of Hurricane Katrina. And she cautions about ignoring the need to be self-sufficient, self-contained, and to accept the possibility that you will be on your own.

"The reality is that we all are subject to some kind of disaster. . . . To ignore that fact is short-sighted. If you want to make it through and have your sanity at the end of the disaster, you need to be at least apprised a little bit, or be aware of the reality that the universe is not going to rescue you if there is a big disaster. You need to be able to be self-sufficient. Everybody needs to do that. It's shocking, in Louisiana, the number of people who don't know where the turnoff valve for their gas is. The one thing I learned in California is that you are ready all the time, you know where the turnoff valve is, and you expect no help to be there. Here, it is, 'Why aren't you helping me now?' That is unrealistic and impossible."

Four years post-Katrina, she feels that she is in better physical shape. Every day, she runs 4 miles, and she goes regularly to the gym. "I thought if there is going to be another storm, I need to be in shape if

I am going to deal with that again. I am going to have to prepare and I will be ready for that potential because I live in a place where hurricanes hit. I have to come to grips with that reality."

Cheryl Martin

I knew when everybody else had family to hold on to, I had my furry little friends to hold on to. I was not about to let them perish.

Cheryl Martin, RN, grew up in upstate New York, in the small city of Amsterdam. A graduate of Albany Medical Center in New York, she came to New Orleans on October 26, 1983, as a traveling nurse. She worked medical/surgical and oncology. In 2000, she joined the staff at Lindy Boggs Medical Center as a nursing supervisor.

On Saturday, August 27, Cheryl had no idea what awaited her at work. She remembers fielding calls from over a dozen staffers who called in to say they were sick or evacuating because of the storm. She did not leave the hospital until 10 o'clock that evening "because of the volume of calls and my desire to try and leave the night supervisor in better shape. It was futile. Nursing agencies that usually were able to provide some assistance were canceling their personnel."

By the time she returns home, she learns more about the pending storm. She recalls "a bad feeling came over her." Her neighbor, Miss Elizabeth, knocks on her door to tell her that she is leaving for Mississippi with her son. Cheryl's neighbor had always taken care of her pets whenever Cheryl had to work for a storm. Now Miss Elizabeth is leaving and can not take Cheryl's two dogs and four cats.

"She wanted me to go with her, but she could not take my pets. I had to work, but I could not leave my furry family. Miss Elizabeth refused to evacuate unless I could be at work and bring my animals. I called the chief nursing officer. She said I could bring them if they were in pet carriers."

Within hours after ending her weekend shift, Cheryl is returning to the hospital, driving against the mass exodus of cars heading away from New Orleans. "They must have thought, 'What is this fool doing going the wrong way?'" she smiles.

She settles her brood on the first floor by the physical therapy area and reports to work. Early Monday, the hurricane comes through. Some windows shatter from the storm pressure. "You could hear the popping sound as windows blew out," she says. "Then you had to wait until the wind sucked back out before you could open the door and enter a room. Patients were moved into the hallways to protect them from glass debris, wind, and rain. They looked so frightened. The staff did an excellent job of trying to reassure them. I went in and out of patients' rooms, singing. I made up jingles for the patients. I received grateful smiles in return. I tried to make sure they saw me with a smile and something pleasant to say. It was my effort to calm them and maybe help get them more relaxed. You could see the fear and uncertainty in so many faces."

As the floodwaters rose in the Mid-City neighborhood, several residents seek refuge at the hospital, which has lost generator power because of the flooding. The new arrivals are housed on the second floor. The second floor and above are occupied by patients, employees, and family members. One of the hospital operators becomes distressed when she looks out of a window and sees her son clinging to a chain link fence, water up to his chin. He is trying to reach the hospital. Cheryl remembers a woman who arrived by the ER ramp, experiencing chest pains.

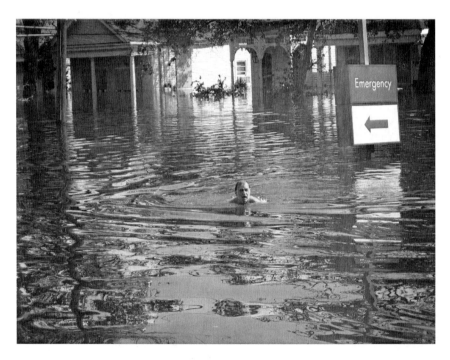

A man swims through the flooded Mid-City area of New Orleans to reach the Lindy Boggs Medical Center's emergency entrance on Bienville Street. Photo by Pablo Moncada.

"There was nothing we could do other than treat her symptoms, maybe give her a little pain medicine," explains Cheryl. "I had to tell the family member that we had no services to be able to provide for her. And what broke my heart was when I told them there wasn't much that we could do, and he said, 'Well, that's OK. I think she would rather be at home.' And I watched him go away in the boat with her. To this day, I still wonder, did she survive? Did they make it out? Was it just anxiety causing her symptoms?"

Cheryl says she never felt in jeopardy at the hospital. "I felt that I was going to be OK. A fireman from a local firehouse had a bunch of dogs that he brought to us. When he left to return to his group, he left me his gun. But I felt comfortable, with my 80-pound Catahoula and the fact that the other people were there. I heard all bad kinds of things were happening. I could see the fires. It was kind of hard at night because you could hear people screaming for help inside their homes or from the rooftops. And there was nothing you could do to help them. What could you do? You couldn't get to them. You couldn't get them to come to you. Then one day, all of these helicopters appeared, lowering their baskets to rescue people."

Cheryl helps patients evacuate from the hospital. She injures her leg when she slips on loose rocks on the hospital roof. When the first responders arrive at the hospital, Cheryl says they did field triage. The frailest of the patients are brought to one section on the east side of the hospital, where a few staff members stay and take care of them, until a medical evacuation transport can move them. As the last group of hospital employees evacuates, Cheryl opts to stay. She promises her colleagues that she will help take care of their pets.

"I had no family. I had no idea if I had a home," she says. "I absolutely knew I had lost my car and my job. My friends were scattered all over the country, and who knew when we were going to see one another. I knew, when everybody else had family to hold on to, I had my furry little friends to hold on to. I was not about to let them perish. I made a decision that we could stay until the other patients and then the pets could get out."

Also staying behind with Cheryl to help take care of the eight critically ill patients are two physicians, a respiratory therapist, a chaplain, and another nurse. Alone in the hospital, they collect the canned goods, radios, flashlights, and batteries and store them in the area where they are staying. Cheryl recalls they were unable to lock the hospital's front doors and improvised by tying oxygen tubing to secure them. They wanted to deter anyone trying to break into the hospital. "I became frightened when the firemen left," says Cheryl. "I had felt so much more secure with their presence, but now they were gone."

There is an eerie quiet in the cavernous hospital as Cheryl walks the floors. The hallways, which had been filled with people, are now still. Linens are strewn on beds. Sleeping bags are rolled up in a corner. Vending machines are stripped of their contents. The Command Center in administration is no longer the center of activity and communications.

That evening, Cheryl checks on the pets. She has kept her pets on the third floor. A few others are in administration. The majority are on the fifth floor, which, years ago, had been used as a psychiatric unit. It has access to a sheltered area on the roof. On the fifth floor, she discovers that one of the dogs has died from the stress of the storm. She also finds a Chihuahua in a laundry basket. It has just given birth.

"Through nursing all the years you say, 'With life comes death and with death comes life.' And I got an opportunity to see it," she says.

Another group of rescuers arrive at the hospital before 24 hours has passed. This time, they are there to vacate the last of the hospital employees.

Cheryl describes one of the rescuers: "this gigantic man. He must have been 6 foot 6. He was huge, and he had just as much weaponry around his body as his size. He pointed to me and said, 'You, you are an employee. You have to leave.' And I looked at him and said, 'OK, I quit.'"

The man seems stunned by her reply. Then one physician turns to Cheryl and tells her to go. He will stay. Because he is not a hospital employee, he says they cannot make him leave. The two make a pact that Cheryl will do what she needs to do on the outside, while he does what he needs to do on the inside. A tearful Cheryl leaves. She is air-evacuated to a sister hospital located north of Lake Pontchartrain in Slidell. Arriving at the hospital, she recalls a company public relations staffer who promised her that as soon as the last of the people were evacuated from Lindy Boggs Medical Center, they would contact Oprah Winfrey to see about helping with the animal rescue.

"When I left the building, I grabbed the wrong bag. I was distressed because I was leaving my animals. I had no money, no cell phone charger, no credit cards, nothing. I had none of my important papers, so I went off on my own when I got to the hospital and sat away from everybody. A woman started talking with me. She said that she had a sister, Cheryl, who worked at the Whitney Bank near the hospital. She later brought me to the bank and helped me access my account until I could get back on the south shore and get established."

With no place to go and part of the city still flooded, Cheryl stays at the north shore hospital. When the animals are evacuated from Lindy Boggs Medical Center, they are brought to the hospital before continuing to a veterinarian in Hattiesburg, Mississippi. Cheryl's reunion with her pets is joyful, but brief. When it is time to part, she volunteers to accompany all of the animals to Mississippi.

"I jumped on the bus," she says. "I had so many animals trying to get close to me because they had been separated from regular human contact for several days. During the ride I broke up a fight between two dogs. There was another dog that had been leashed to its seat. But when it slipped off the seat, it almost strangled. I am glad that I was there."

From Mississippi, the animals were transported to a veterinarian in Toledo, Texas, who raised $12,000 and acquired a van and volunteers to assist with animal rescue post–Hurricane Katrina. Later she reconnects with her neighbor Miss Elizabeth, who drives Cheryl to Texas, where they meet with the volunteers. One of Cheryl's cats is lost in the hospital but, nearly 2 months later, is found. Of the 41 dogs, 16 cats, and 2 gerbils that had been housed at Lindy Boggs Medical Center, Cheryl says only one animal was not returned to its owner because he could not be located. When Cheryl returns to NorthShore Regional Medical Center, she volunteers again.

"I had the opportunity to ride on a Black Hawk. They evacuated 12 people from an assisted-living center, and I went. When we returned to the hospital, they gave me some of their military shirts. They hugged me and thanked me for my service. I said 'No, I thank you for yours.' What they had done I think was absolutely amazing. The military was wonderful."

Cheryl needs to find a way to get back to her home. She finds it through a Kraft Foods vendor she meets in the hospital cafeteria. He tells her that volunteers are needed to help give out food to the military who are working near the breached 17th Street Canal in Metairie. Cheryl volunteers, and minutes later is in a van crossing the Causeway Bridge across Lake Pontchartrain. Once in Metairie, she stays for a few weeks at a local pastor's residence.

"For several weeks, I didn't know if I had a house. I had lost my car and this was an answer to getting back near my home. When we were driving through the areas that had flooded, it was surreal. There were buses and cars on the wrong side of the street, clothing on the overpasses, trees on the telephone poles. On the Causeway we were driving on the wrong side of the bridge, zigzagging in and out of debris. I have photos of a boat on top of a house. When I returned to my neighborhood, it looked like a war zone. There wasn't a bit of greenery and everything was brown.

"I saw my neighbors and other elderly people who had stayed. I am not a creature of change. After Katrina, I needed the stability of my house—my little environment that I was familiar with, without having to change to another place."

Hurricane Katrina also taught her an important lesson. "All those things I had before is just stuff. I had a vast collection of art. I didn't know if I had a house and I didn't care about any of that. Later, when I left my house for Hurricane Gustav, I said, 'This storm can take it.' Because you know what? It is just stuff."

For the next 5 months, Cheryl works as a volunteer. She helps her friends gut their office building destroyed by the storm. She accompanies her elderly neighbors and stands in line for distribution of water and meals ready to eat (MREs), calling it "the most humbling experience of my life. I have worked since I was 13 years old and no one has ever given me anything. So to have to be at the mercy of the public and see just how devastating it was for people, it was sad."

On January 20, 2007, Cheryl returns to nursing. She sees marked improvements at area hospitals for storm preparation. "For Katrina, I don't think hospitals were given enough advanced knowledge to be able to evacuate. When you are preparing late Saturday and early Sunday for something that is coming Monday morning, I think that's a little bit too late."

Before Hurricane Gustav makes landfall on September 1, 2008, Cheryl is the night shift nursing supervisor at a New Orleans–area hospital and receives a phone call from Homeland Security. A representative wants to know about the fuel supply at her hospital. She relays the information, and by midnight, a tanker arrives to bring additional fuel for the facility's generators.

"The next day I got another phone call," adds Cheryl. "They called to see how everything was. I later heard on the news about the evacuation of those facilities whose generators had failed. Fuel was brought to the open hospitals to make sure their generators worked, so they could take the evacuated patients. That never happened for Katrina."

Cheryl no longer has her dogs. One that had been ill for years died. The companion dog followed 18 months later. She has the four cats, which stay at home when she works for a pending storm. Many hospitals have policies that prevent employees from bringing their pets with them when they work for storms. Four years post-Katrina, Cheryl says support from other states is still needed.

"They can help us hold the government accountable. What's to say that another major event won't hit their area. It's the same thing. Everybody across the country gets hit with something somewhere. In California its wildfires, in Oklahoma its tornadoes, Louisiana it's hurricanes. If we don't hold the government accountable and step things up to protect our environment, to protect our homes, then we are going to have some serious problems. They need to know. They need to be aware that this is happening and also about the humanity, the wonderful outpouring of help from people that is still happening in this area. I think people finally did realize what happened here."

Lois Spengeman

Everything that was battery operated eventually died. There were no monitors. Just wetting a patient's lips, using a wet compress to give relief from the heat—we tried to take care of people in the most humane way possible.

Lois Spengeman, RN, BSN, MHCM, received her basic nursing training through the Louisiana State University (LSU) associate degree nursing program after completing a degree in anthropology and art history at Newcomb College. She later went on to pursue a bachelor of science degree in nursing at Loyola and a master's degree in health care management at the University of New Orleans (UNO). After graduating from LSU, she went to work full-time at Southern Baptist Hospital on a medical/surgical floor. About a year later, she transferred to the postanesthesia care unit (PACU), and worked there for many years. As the hospital changed hands several times and there was restructuring of nursing departments, Lois was afforded leadership opportunities in management, becoming head nurse of first one area, and then several. At the time of Katrina, Lois was the director of surgical services at Lindy Boggs Medical Center, which included surgery, PACU, ambulatory care, endoscopy, and central sterile.

On Friday, August 26, Lois Spengeman joins a group of her friends for dinner. News of a negative biopsy report for one of them was cause for celebration. When the dinner conversation turns to the question of where everyone had hotel reservations in preparation of the coming hurricane, Lois says that was the first time she heard that the storm was headed their way.

The next day, she is at Lindy Boggs Medical Center for a prestorm meeting and preparations. On Sunday, at two o'clock in the afternoon, she reports to work, while her husband, 10-year-old daughter, and their two dogs are on their way to her mother's home in Vicksburg, Mississippi. At her home, a few miles from the hospital, they had left two cats with what they thought would be enough food until they returned.

Lois calls in teams for all areas except ambulatory care. Friday is the last day for surgeries, and physicians had begun discharging as many patients as possible before the weekend.

Lois says Sunday evening was a relatively quiet time at the hospital where staff, families of patients, and employees and pets were now housed. Recalls Lois, "We all thought we were so good about letting people bring pets. After that storm, I thought, 'No pets, ever.' It was horrible after so many days."

That evening is standard routine for the staff, who check supplies of water and batteries. Central service staff move equipment from the basement to upstairs. The phone service works throughout the night. There are small groups of visitors who pass the time watching movies. Others call their friends and family members who had evacuated the city. Lois reaches her husband and daughter to tell them all is well—she will call them again after the storm. As she makes room in her office to sleep, Lois can hear the winds and the breaking of windows as the hurricane comes through. One side of the hospital reports loss of power. The backup generators start humming.

On Monday morning, there is relief among everyone that the storm has caused no major damage. Lois's staff make rounds to each floor, checking to see if anyone needs to take a break or replenish their water or other supplies.

"Everybody was so thankful we had made it through the storm," says Lois. "It was sunshine outside. The patients are fine. Everybody is greatly relieved. We couldn't do anything about leaving yet, but everything was in good shape. The staff is sitting out on the emergency ramp, playing guitars and singing. And phone service was working. I was able to call Vicksburg. I told them, 'See you in a couple of days.'"

And then the water comes. Standing next to her coworkers at the hospital's entrance facing South Jefferson Davis Parkway, Lois says, they watch it rise.

"Our chief nursing officer said she had been watching that water and says it's not going down. Others started to take note," she relays. "We watched the water level on a column and pretty soon it was evident it was coming up. Soon cars were flooded and people were wading through this water, trying to come to the hospital."

The water pours over the hospital's floodgates and into the basement. Phone lines are out. The Command Post is set up, where staff can get updates on the hospital's status. Inside the hospital, Lois says she feels protected, but the unknown elements outside "were the frightening part. Nobody knew really anything what was happening outside."

As the waters fill the basement, the backup generators stop. The interior of the hospital is dark.

"We all kicked into gear trying to set up hygienic restrooms, start rationing water, and looking at food supplies," says Lois. "There was an industrious group in the maintenance department. They found a boat and

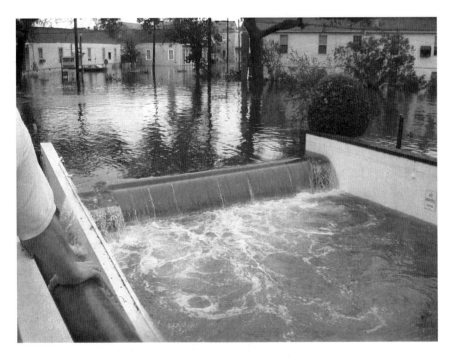

Like a waterfall, flood waters cascade over a barrier to the loading dock of Lindy Boggs Medical Center. The waters flooded the hospital basement, which housed supplies and equipment, the kitchen, the pharmacy, and the morgue. Photo by Pablo Moncada.

started shuttling people who were coming from the community to dry ground by Delgado University because we didn't want to bring them into the hospital and compromise even more of our resources. The maintenance guys also went to the adjacent medical office building, where they got antibiotics from the physician offices. Once we lost battery power, we quickly realized there was nothing we could save in surgery. We started thinking how we could prevent the walls from sweating and prevent everything from being contaminated. But after a while, we realized there was really nothing we could do."

Patients in the ER are moved to the second-floor PACU. In the windowless PACU, nurses tend to the patients, using flashlights as their only source of illumination.

"Everything that was battery operated eventually died," says Lois. "There were no monitors. Just wetting a patient's lips, using a wet compress to give relief from the heat—we tried to take care of people in the most humane way possible."

In her 25 years of nursing, Lois never imagined working conditions without electricity or running water.

"MASH units in third world countries probably have some sort of clinic operation set up. They may not meet our standards, but at that point we were just sort of swinging by the seat of our pants. We just didn't have the tools that you would normally fall back on. You had no chart, no computer. It was all gone. But at the same time there were a lot of patients who were survivors. They worked with us and we worked with them, and most of them got out. But at what price? Every hospital experienced death."

As the temperature climbs inside the hospital, Lois checks on her staff to ensure that they are not succumbing to heat and dehydration. By Tuesday, there are some family members and staff who feel claustrophobic in the confines of the hospital.

"There was a period where people went into stress overload and their memory was not clear. Talking to the employees between Tuesday and Wednesday, some of them didn't remember if they ate or drank, or how much, or if they used the restroom," she adds.

"There was a really good team effort. Everybody pulled together and protected each other and befriended people that maybe they weren't very close to on a day-to-day basis because it was a smaller group. There was that feeling that we just need to get through this, we are all going to be OK. Certainly help will be here.

"Even though there were some emotional times where people would get frightened or upset about something, I felt everybody was pretty much in there for the long haul and to support each other and stay to the end."

When help arrives from the Shreveport Fire Department, the employees form a fire brigade going down the dark stairwells to bring the patients to the first floor, where boats wait for them. A small group of the most critically ill patients cannot be evacuated with the others. A handful of medical and nursing staff remains.

Looking back on those days at Lindy Boggs Medical Center, Lois says, there is value in having others understand the challenges the staff faced. "There are a lot of things that you never think about until you are put into that situation. And when you are, all of a sudden you realize how important certain things are in terms of preparation or planning. For me, I would say no animals. Even though a lot of people I know feel very strongly that they wouldn't leave their animals, I think they would have to go to the next tier. You make arrangements ahead of time because quickly, what used to be so acceptable with the dogs and cats, all of a sudden it is, 'Oh, my gosh, we don't need anything extra.' There were extra family members of patients and employees. We had one incident where an employee brought to the hospital a family member who needed medical care because of a chronic condition. She thought the hospital was the safest place to bring her loved one. Well, it didn't turn out that way at all, because we couldn't provide treatment, and when systems gave out, it was really frightening. He needed dialysis. We had great concerns, he got to a clinic in Lake Charles, Louisiana. You may think you are a good employer by allowing your staff to bring in family members, but you realize the extra liability you have in doing so. I think in a true emergency, you just need your essential personnel."

On Wednesday, August 31, around 6:00 P.M., Lois evacuates with her colleagues. A boat ferries the hospital evacuees to the nearby post office. From there, they are directed to an army helicopter.

"They pack us in like sardines," she says. "The doors remain open, giving us an interesting view during the flight."

They are brought to the Interstate 10 and Causeway intersection in Metairie. Some of the nurses and physicians go the triage site to offer their assistance. "There were masses of people. The entire scene was chaotic," says Lois. "It was hard to tell who was in charge. That's when you had the feeling things were out of control. I wouldn't say I feared for my life. It wasn't dangerous that way. But we as a group formed a circle around the children because there was a lot of drinking going on from the community members. There were piles of MREs, and water that you helped yourself to. One of our doctors tried to negotiate a bus for the Lindy Boggs employees. He stayed behind and worked at the MASH area. He must have been successful because we finally got on a bus."

The bus is to take them to Lake Charles, Louisiana. However, the employees persuade the driver to drive to Baton Rouge. There they connect with an employee's relatives, who open their home for the evacuees. It is midnight when Lois calls her husband. He drives to Baton Rouge to get her.

Since Lindy Boggs Medical Center is now closed, Lois's next job is as a case manager at a New Orleans hospital.

"I feel like I am in a transitional place, and I haven't really decided what direction I want to go," she offers. "I am enjoying my current work because I am still involved with the doctors and patients. I am learning the criteria of the insurance side, because when you are at the bedside you don't pay much attention to that. So that part is interesting because it's different. It's definitely a different pace."

Four years later, Lois finds many of her friends and former colleagues "still evolving. From where they were they may not have found that next niche. Others may have found it and are happy, but they made a lot of changes getting there. And then there are some people who are still not sure."

Linda van Dyke

Some of us went to the roof. We wrote on sheets—NEED PATIENTS OUT. We hoped someone would see us and realize we were a hospital.

Linda Van Dyke, RN, began working at 18 at Chalmette General Hospital, where she worked as a nursing assistant and a unit secretary, until she graduated as a licensed practical nurse (LPN). She then began working at Southern Baptist Hospital where she continued her nursing education and in 1990 graduated from LSU Medical Center. She is married to Kevin Burge and has one son, Paul.

Linda Van Dyke started her nursing career as an LPN in 1982. She joined the ER staff at Lindy Boggs Medical Center, which at the time was called Mercy campus of Memorial Medical Center. Having worked at the hospital for several storms before, she felt that the one named Katrina would not be any different from the others.

But just in case this is the "big one," she wants the ER to have adequate staffing, and she makes sure that her 20-year-old son and mother are far away from the metro New Orleans area.

"If this was the big one, I would have enough to do and wanted them safe and away. We might have a lot of devastation, damage, flooding, but I never imagined that amount of flooding," she says. Friday, August 26, she works her 7:00 A.M. to 7:00 P.M. shift. Linda offers to help the new unit director call the staff who will be on weekend assignment.

"We told them to bring their 3-day supply of clothes and food," she recounts. "At the time, we had weekend nurses that were scheduled to work Saturday and Sunday. I told them to be prepared to stay because they may not get to leave. We had the largest turnout of staff in the ER."

Ending her Saturday shift, Linda returns to her home in Norco, west of New Orleans. Her husband, Kevin, has already gone to work. He is an EMT. Linda will bring their pet Labrador retriever with her to the hospital.

"Sunday we were deciding how many we needed for each shift. We were holding admits in the ER and the hospital was full. People were still coming in, being admitted as seen," she says. "As we had seen for other storms, we had cases of families dropping off their parent with a suitcase and then driving off. Someone came in needing dialysis, concerned they were not going to be able to get it once the storm hits. For storms we expected a full house."

The hospital goes on ambulance diversion, with cases redirected to other area hospitals with available patient beds, but ambulances continue to arrive at Lindy Boggs's ER. By Sunday night, all nine ER beds are taken.

"We had enough staff but were praying no more patients who needed critical care would come by ambulance because we were already holding two critical patients in the ER. We had received one nursing home patient and another patient who came to the lobby in a wheelchair and on oxygen."

Those two patients are assigned to Linda. By the time her shift ends at 7:00 P.M., activity in the ER has quieted. Linda remains on the unit until midnight, reviewing the census and planning for the next day. She and other ER staffers set up sleeping quarters on the fourth floor in the transplant unit. Linda calls her son and tells him, "So far so good, getting hot, the wind is bad, but we're OK."

Sleep is fleeting for Linda as she listens to the wind howl and the windows breaking. Around midnight, the hospital loses electricity. The hum of generators can be heard. Linda checks on her dog in his kennel on the hospital roof. She is told that her dog barked incessantly, until she became hoarse. Later, when the pharmacist asks Linda if she can bring her dog in at night to guard the pharmacy, which was relocated to the nurse's station on the fourth floor, Linda is only too happy to oblige.

By Monday morning, the storm has passed. Then the heat comes. Patients are in their gowns, but the staff remove their socks and sheets in their efforts to keep them cool. At the start of her shift, Linda has a few minutes to step outside and check on her car. There is standing water in the parking lot, but nothing of consequence. Before her shift ends, the situation changes. Flooding is reported. No one knows the source.

People were still coming to the hospital. "We did not turn them away. They had no place to go," says Linda. "At one point we put them in the waiting area, but after a while, we couldn't hold anybody, so we had them stay outside by the ER ramp. Everybody worked together, and we had the unit secretary, who worked every day."

As the water makes it way up the ER ramp, the decision is made to move vertically. "There was a rumor there was going to be more surge and an additional 16 feet of water," says Linda. "I don't know where that came from, but we had no outside communications. The water was already flooding the basement and topping the barrier they had set up there. You could see the water moving up the ER ramp."

Firemen who stayed at the hospital during the storm help move the nine patients to the second floor. Linda reassures the patients and their families that the move is for safety reasons. "I told them everything would be all right, before you know it, we will be out of here. Somebody will come evacuate us. We don't expect to be here very long," she says.

On the second floor, the expansive recovery unit is converted for ER use, but there are no windows in the unit. Linda says that presented its own challenges. "You work 12 hours and have no daylight," she explains. "No windows meant it was pitch dark if you did not have a flashlight. And when you finished working, it was dark outside. You were in constant darkness."

Knowing that it is two flights up to reach the pharmacy and two flights down to retrieve supplies from the ER, Linda determines which stairwell gives her the quickest access. Using a flashlight, she feels her way along the stairwell walls and steps. This is no time to fall.

"When we moved to recovery, there was no way we could set up triage the way we wanted to," explains Linda. "We stayed there Tuesday, then decided we had to relocate. It was too hot and we had no natural light during the day."

Some patients whose conditions had improved since their arrival are given discharge orders and released from the ER. They move to the second floor. Downstairs, water laps at the top of the ER ramp. The staff resituates its unit in the west wing by Dialysis. One room is set up for triage. In their new location, broken windows usher in a welcome breeze. Windows that do not open are broken to help with cross-ventilation. The ER staff are notified that some people have become ill. Their symptoms are nausea, vomiting, and diarrhea. The situation is monitored.

"Before the hurricane, we had discussed hygiene and sanitation measures—what to do about changing linens, keeping patients cool and hydrated," says Linda. "We had a plan for human waste disposal. We did everything we could to bag and double-bag everything, and used every storage capacity available. If we had stayed any longer than we did at the hospital, it would have been a nightmare.

"There was no problem having enough nurses," she continues. "We did rounds with the physicians to see all the patients. We assessed who still needed oxygen because we were being told the oxygen force was going out and medicines were becoming depleted. We discussed all of these issues. It was well done. We took it day by day."

Only a few become ill. There are no trauma cases. The staff treats cuts and abrasions on several of the people who have made their way through the water to reach the hospital. One of them is a paramedic with Orleans Parish. He has walked through waist-high, murky water from Moss Street to bring a generator to the hospital.

It is Tuesday, and Day 3 for Linda at the hospital. In the morning, a group of employees gather with one of the hospital chaplains, for a moment of prayer. Then they review that day's agenda. It is hot. People are hungry. Food is emptied from ice chests and refrigerators. "We were rationing. We had cereal. Peanut butter. But you didn't feel like eating. It was too hot. By Tuesday, I was getting tired because you are not sleeping at night. There is the constant noise of the helicopters. We saw the Coast Guard landing on the American Can Company near the hospital. There were a whole bunch of people on the condominium's roof. Our command center tells us the Coast Guard knows we are at the hospital. They could not tell us when rescue would come. Some of us went to the

hospital roof. We wrote on sheets—NEED PATIENTS OUT. We hoped someone would see us and realize we were a hospital."

Helicopters land and evacuees board them. It is like a choreographed
air ballet; as one helicopter lifts off, another one lands. The grassy area
by the post office is one block away from the hospital, yet it seems so far
away to Linda and others at Lindy Boggs.

"At night we could hear people calling out for help," she says. "It was
terrible. You couldn't see where the cries were coming from. You couldn't
see who it was. It seemed to never stop. And we could see the fires
downtown. We were worried about fire because we had no alarms."

On Wednesday, August 31, help arrives. Linda is assigned to make
rounds with the Shreveport Fire Department. Floor by floor, she escorts
them as the firemen determine each person's level for evacuation. In less
than 2 hours, rounds are completed. "We did whatever they told us to
do. They wasted no time, and we listened. We gave them our attention.

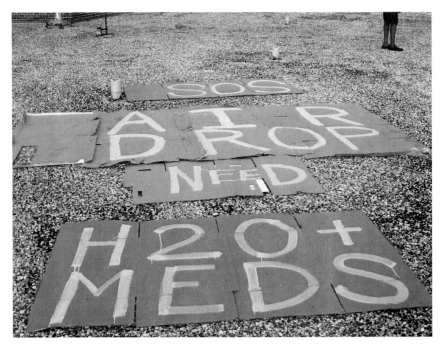

On the roof of Lindy Boggs Medical Center, a cardboard SOS sign made by hospital
employees attempts to get the attention of the helicopter crews that conducted search
and rescue missions following Hurricane Katrina. Photo by Pablo Moncada.

We followed their directions. They were very organized, very professional. And the response of the staff was great," Linda says. She pauses. "When they told us there were some people they were not going to take because they were in the most critical condition and fragile, that was very hard for the staff."

The evacuation staging area is at the hospital's loading dock. Engineering and security personnel ferry patients, family members, and staff from the hospital to the grassy area by the post office. Linda says it did not matter which staff member went, as long as the patients got to the patch of green. By early evening, the majority of the patients have been evacuated. Then the rescue stops. "Then it was night. We were told to 'line up against the wall, we are going to make an announcement. Somebody will come and get you tomorrow at daybreak,'" she says. "The Shreveport Fire Department was telling us they have to stop, can't move at night. It is not safe. We didn't know they were getting shot at. We didn't know people were resorting to violence. We didn't know what was going on outside. We got very anxious. We didn't want to spend another night. If there was a fire in the hospital, we had no alarms. We had been told the levees broke, but we didn't know where. We knew the metro area had flooded. We were hoping they would come back but tried not to get our hopes up too high because they were evacuating so many other places."

Linda's dog is moved to the fifth floor, along with other pets. She cannot bear to check on her, knowing the storm and confinement have caused extreme stress for the animal. That evening, few people sleep. In the hallway, a small table is set up. Linda takes out a deck of cards she had brought. They play cards. "We couldn't sleep," offers Linda. "We had to do something to keep our minds occupied. We had a battery-operated radio and sometimes got a Baton Rouge station. My last communications with my family was Sunday night." At four o'clock Thursday morning, they line up in the hallway by the lobby on the first floor of the hospital. They are ready to leave.

"We are not going to eat. We are not going to drink. We don't want to have to use the bathroom," recalls Linda. "There are about 80 of us. Nobody showed up at daybreak. We waited and waited. It was almost noon. I think we decided at that point we didn't know what to do. Nobody was coming to get us. Helicopters are landing on the green patch. There were hundreds of people out there. So the maintenance crew took their boat and brought chairs and rope to the grassy area. They roped off a section just for us and then brought us there. We thought if we were out there in one large group, someone would see us and come. You had to get in the water to get in the boat and out of the boat. You are hot and stinky. Then you stand there in the hot baking sun and just wait."

Finally, the helicopters start landing. Linda's group is taken to the Louis Armstrong International Airport, where Federal Emergency Management Agency personnel think they are the relief workers. Linda tells herself that they must be kidding. They are directed upstairs to an area near a row of closed gift shops. They sit on the floor, while throngs of people mill about. A woman in a Delta Airlines uniform walks over to Linda and her colleagues. She tells them a cargo plane has dropped supplies from Atlanta. The plane is returning to Atlanta. Do they want to take it? "I said, 'I will go anywhere,'" shares Linda. "We were near the gate for the plane and were told to make sure we were in this line with the first hundred people. It was not an organized line. It got wild. People tried to push us out of the way. There were a lot of overhead announcements about firearms, and warnings that you would be arrested if you got on a plane with a gun. We were really worried about that. I was wondering if some people were going to get violent. There was a lot of pushing and shoving. No one seemed to be organizing us. We held hands. We were not going to be split up."

When Linda and two fellow nurses arrive in Atlanta, Delta buses are waiting to bring them to a Holiday Inn. They are given vouchers for room service, hats, and t-shirts. Linda and her coworker share a room. They call their families. Linda reaches her husband. For 5 days, neither has known if the other was safe. The following morning, Delta Airlines offers them free flights to wherever they need to go. An airline representative gets their tickets and boarding passes and escorts them to the gate. Linda takes the flight to Baton Rouge, where her family is waiting. "On the flight home, I am thinking I will never see my dog again. I don't know if I will ever do this again. I know I have no job, no car, and perhaps no home," she says. "When I got to Baton Rouge, Kevin met me. He was working with a police officer. When the flooding started they went to a hospital on the West Bank. I did not realize how bad everything was until I had left. We had one day together and then he had to return to New Orleans for work."

Her family is safe, and Linda is told that the pets at Lindy Boggs may be at a shelter in Baton Rouge. She has no luck there or at an animal shelter in Gonzalez. She returns home. The hurricane has spared it. Then one night, she receives a phone call from a colleague. The pets are on their way to Texas. If she can leave now and drive to Monroe,

Louisiana, she can claim her dog. Linda drives 6 hours to Monroe and is reunited with her pet. Filthy and several pounds thinner, she needs much coaxing to get into the car.

A month after the storm, Linda returns to emergency care nursing. She is a charge nurse on the night shift. The next hurricane season, for Hurricane Gustav, she is on Team B. She plans to be on the activation team for future storms. She believes opportunity will always be there for improvements and to learn from those who experienced Hurricane Katrina firsthand. "Something like this will happen again—and how better to learn than from those who had been through it, those who know the advantages, the disadvantages, what things they would have done differently?" she asks.

"Some people tell me they know what we dealt with, but their ER was closed and they didn't have patients. They were not there for days. They had the power for small air-conditioning units and fans, so they weren't hot. They talk about people not getting along. I am thinking, what? We never had that. Nobody argued. We had a total, cohesive, cooperative group that was open to all suggestions and that made suggestions. We shared whatever we had with each other. I still am in touch with them and miss them.

"If I had a choice, I think I wouldn't want to do it again. But then again, this is who I am. I can't imagine not being involved and helping people. Now knowing what I went through, maybe I do have a lot more to offer than others that didn't have this experience. So I need to be available. There are some who are listening. If anything, I can bring to the table a lot of suggestions and a lot of things we did that maybe will be helpful to those in administration and upper management because they have never been through it. They need to be well prepared. Before we evacuated, we talked about going to an 8-hour shift, instead of a 12-hour shift—restructuring the shift so we could address some of the anxiety and fatigue people experienced. I know I could bring my experience to those who never had to do this."

4 Memorial Medical Center

From its opening in 1926 as Southern Baptist Hospital, Memorial Medical Center would come to care for generations of families from throughout the New Orleans area and beyond. In the course of its history, it would change ownership three times and also undergo subsequent name changes and attempts to rebrand its identity in the community. Yet despite these changes, the Southern Baptist Hospital association never faded (Greene, 1976).

Eleven years before the Baptist missionaries opened the hospital on property donated by the citizens of New Orleans, the Southern Baptist Convention began addressing the need for hospitals at their 1915 convention, when they formed the Southern Baptist Hospital Conference. Two years later, a committee on hospitals was appointed. When their 1917 convention was hosted in New Orleans, the idea of building a hospital in New Orleans was put forth by Clementine Morgan Kelly, a missionary who worked there tending to the infirm in hospital charity wards and the homeless on the streets of the city (Greene, 1976).

By 1920, there were 1,554 hospital beds in New Orleans. The demand called for at least 4,000 beds (Greene, 1976). In addition to the steady stream of patients from the greater New Orleans area and communities of south Louisiana, families from Latin America also came to the Crescent City for medical treatment. It was in this climate that the Southern Baptist Hospital Conference established a Standing Committee for Hospitals at their convention. After assessing a location for the hospital site, the committee would later report,

> A very desirable site consisting of two entire city blocks has been decided upon for the location of the institution provided title to the property can be conveyed in the manner satisfactory to the Home Mission Board. The Association of Commerce of New Orleans proposes to present this site to the Board and the matter is now pending between the Home Mission Board and the Association of Commerce. It is the earnest hope of your committee that this seriously important matter and wonderful opportunity shall continue to be handled with all possible wisdom and dispatch to the end that Southern Baptists shall, in the not distant future, erect in the Crescent City a hospital of such proportions that it shall be at once a stronghold for our cause, a channel of service and blessing, and an adequate expression of our Baptist faith and purpose. (Southern Baptist Convention Annual, 1921, pp. 48–49)

The hospital was built with a fund established with the help of the archbishop of New Orleans and individuals representing all denominations. On Thanksgiving Day, November 24, 1924, groundbreaking ceremonies at the 2700 block of Napoleon Avenue drew over 1,000 attendees.

The hospital grounds would be bordered by Cadiz Street and Clara Street. The eight-story building had three elevators, 16 sun parlors, 28 telephones, a pharmacy, a flower shop, a barbershop, and a vegetable garden on-site. Located in the basement were the kitchen, cafeteria, and dining area. On the first floor were the lobby, waiting rooms, chapel, and administration offices. Bed capacity was 248, including 36 beds in the nursery. The total price tag for the land, construction, and equipment was $1,250,000 (Greene, 1976).

On March 8, 1926, when the hospital officially opened its doors, there were 100 employees. Many of them would remain on staff for more than 30 years. By the end of the inaugural year, there had been 4,414 admits and 291 births (Greene, 1976). In 1926 and 1927, flooding dumped 7 feet of water into the hospital, disrupting services. Flooding would continue to be an issue for the hospital during tropical storms and hurricanes, as the hospital site rested on one of the lowest elevations in the New Orleans area. Not to be deterred by the threat of flooding, the hospital stored boats on-site, which were used to ferry patients and staff from nearby higher ground to the hospital when heavy rainfall made the hospital an island.

As the New Orleans population grew, Southern Baptist Hospital added additional wings and, by fall 1940, had 364 beds. That year, a plasma bank was established in the pathology department, becoming the first laboratory in Louisiana and one of the first in the country equipped for processing plasma by the standards of the National Institutes of Health. In 1956, the hospital celebrated another first—the birth of twins, which were the largest born in the United States and the largest in the annals of medical history at the time. The twin girls weighed a total of nearly 20 pounds (Greene, 1976).

By the 1960s, the hospital had a 640-bed capacity, an extended-care facility, a heliport, an eight-story parking garage, a school of nursing, and a medical office building. By its 40th anniversary in 1966, the hospital had served an estimated 600,000 patients. In September of the following year, the 100,000th baby was born at Southern Baptist Hospital (Greene, 1976).

The next two decades were marked by continued growth of hospital services and third-generation patients choosing Baptist for their treatment. In 1994, Southern Baptist merged with Mercy Hospital, located 5 miles away. Mercy Hospital traced its origin to 1830s Ireland, where Catherine McAuley, an orphan, used an inheritance from her guardian to found the Sisters of Mercy to serve the poor. In 1869, the sisters arrived in New Orleans, opening a school and clinic. The clinic grew to become Mercy Hospital, occupying several locations before moving, in 1953, to Jefferson Davis Parkway and Bienville Street in the Mid-City area of New Orleans, near Bayou St. John.

The merger that created Mercy + Baptist Hospital created the largest private hospital at the time in the New Orleans area, with 726 beds. Management also merged to become Christian Health Ministries, and the two separate medical staffs became one. In 1995, Tenet Healthcare Corporation acquired Mercy + Baptist and, the following year, renamed it Memorial Medical Center, Baptist and Mercy Campuses. In 1998, the two separated to become Memorial Medical Center and Lindy Boggs Medical Center.

In August 2005, Memorial Medical Center was a 315-bed facility with a medical staff of 700 plus and a workforce of 2,500. The nursing staff totaled 900. One of these was Denise Danna, DNS, RN, who started at Memorial in 1973 as a student nurse. "We had the first nurse tech program in the city. In high school, at Sacred Heart on Canal Street, you were required to do community service hours. I joined a few of my friends to volunteer at Charity Hospital. I guess that was the beginning," says Denise.

During her career, Denise rose through the ranks, becoming chief nursing officer at Memorial Medical Center in 1990. At the time, she was working on a master's degree in community health from Louisiana State University (LSU). She would later earn a doctorate in nursing in 1999. During her 32-year tenure at Memorial, she witnessed the ebb and flow of changes as the hospital expanded services and medical staff. She also came to know the heart and soul of the hospital through the men and women who worked there and the patients they served.

Denise was a seasoned veteran of numerous storms. The hurricane season from June 1 to November 30 is one of the most heightened periods for the city's and hospital's emergency preparedness. Tropical depressions, hurricanes, and ground-saturating seasonal rains threatened to cause flooding around the hospital. At the end of summer 1998, Tropical Storm Francis dumped 10 inches of rain in 24 hours on New Orleans. By noon, Cadiz Street, fronting the hospital's main entrance, resembled a flowing river. Waters eventually receded that evening. On September 28, 2 weeks later, Hurricane Georges threatened the area with 110-mph winds, causing a massive evacuation of 1.5 million residents. Georges was the seventh tropical storm, fourth hurricane, and second major hurricane of 1998 for the Atlantic hurricane season.

"For every storm, we had a core team that would report to the hospital and stand in place until all was clear to resume regular services. It is a protocol for emergency preparedness that every hospital follows. But never could I have imagined what Hurricane Katrina would bring," says Denise.

Five nurses recount what they experienced during their last days at Memorial Medical Center during one of the nation's worst disasters. Their stories reveal how remarkable and committed they were as nurses, but how their journey did not end when they were evacuated from the hospital.

Pam Mathews

Nobody should ever have to do this again. No nurse, no patient, no one should ever have to suffer like this.

Pam Mathews, RN, attended LSU Baton Rouge and graduated from the LSU School of Nursing in 1982. In 1981, while she was in nursing school, she started her career at Southern Baptist Hospital in the neonatal intensive care unit (NICU) as a nurse tech and remained there until 2005. During this time, she was employed as a staff nurse, the assistant manager in the NICU, and the manager of the NICU, well-baby nursery, and lactation center. Following Hurricane Katrina, she worked at a law firm reviewing medical records, at the Louisiana Practical Nurse Board of Examiners in the compliance department, and the performance improvement department and as a staff nurse in a local hospital. She is currently employed at LSU Health Sciences Center (LSUHSC) School of Nursing as the student recruiter. Pam has published two articles; one was designated "Article of the Year" by the *American Journal of Maternal/ Child Nursing Clinical* in 2009. She is married and has two children.

On August 27, Katrina moved onshore in south Florida as a Category 1 hurricane and weakened to a tropical storm while over land. As the center moved across Miami-Dade County, Katrina strengthened again to a Category 1 hurricane later that day, when it moved over the eastern Gulf of Mexico. Continuing its southwest direction, Katrina had intensified to a Category 2 hurricane by 11:30 A.M. Eastern Daylight Time on August 26.

On Friday, August 27, the skies are clear in New Orleans. That morning, the Memorial Medical Center Leadership Council meets and reviews the hospital's emergency preparedness plans. The meeting ends with the incident commander informing everyone that they would be called if needed. Pam, a manager of the hospital's NICU for the last 17 years, leaves work feeling the storm will go to Florida.

The next day, the situation changes. Pam lives in the St. Bernard Parish community of Arabi, less than 10 miles from the hospital. Saturday morning, thinking that an evacuation might be ordered, Pam and her daughter Lauren drive to Slidell to retrieve Lauren's car at a local dealership. As they are leaving the house, her son Mat asks her if he would still be able to get his senior class ring that night at his high school, Holy Cross, located in the Ninth Ward.

"I said, 'Maybe you'll get the ring tonight, but if they start evacuating, the dance might be canceled,'" she recalls. By three o'clock that afternoon, her entire family is gone. Her parents, sister, and brother have packed their cars and driven to Houston. They take her two children with them. By midday, Pam is on the phone calling staff who would report to work the next morning as part of Team A. She recalls that Saturday was "a terrible day. I feel like we entered the whole situation fatigued and with some degree of stress because [of] trying to arrange for staffing, by activating Team A and Team B. Team A was the staff who

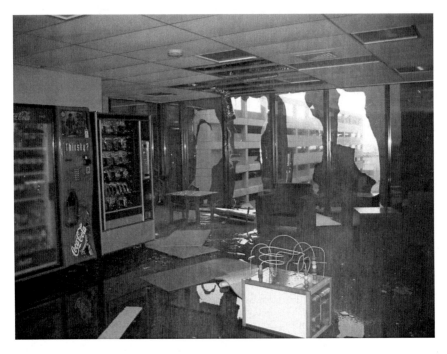

In the women's and infants' waiting area at Memorial Medical Center, Hurricane Katrina winds shattered the floor-to-ceiling windows. Photo by Sandra E. Cordray.

were to work for the emergency and Team B was the relief staff, ready to relieve Team A after 3 days.

"I do feel that I got tremendous cooperation from the staff working on Saturday. . . . I was on the phone constantly, with the phone on one ear, trying to pack my house up, trying to get my family off. Sometimes I had the cell phone and the home phone at the same time, trying to get it all organized. Looking back, I feel like we [the hospital] started out very well organized Sunday morning. Everybody came in according to plan, assignments were made. The care of the patients went very well. I can honestly say I think the patients got, under the circumstances, very good care."

On Sunday, August 28, the women's and infants' division on the sixth floor of the hospital has 50 nurses on duty in the NICU. In the NICU, they have 15 babies, and that night, a neonate transfer comes from University Hospital.

The parents stay in the NICU with their babies. When it is time for evacuation, they are right at their sides. "We didn't separate them, we kept everybody together. We kept them with their babies virtually the whole time," says Pam.

This is not the first storm that Pam has been through at the hospital. "I had been there for all of the hurricanes since I took the management job in 1988 at Memorial. We had always been prepared. The hospital had prepared for the influx of patients, but I don't think we prepared for the exodus of an entire hospital. We had never prepared for that. And I can tell you right now that if I were to do a drill in a hospital setting now, I would have a whole different attitude. The drills were exercises that did not have any reality attached to them. Never, never, ever in my wildest dreams, even walking in there that Sunday morning, I never expected the outcome to be what it was. It never even crossed my mind."

She expects some significant damage from the storm, but nothing of major consequence. It becomes surreal when she receives the continuous e-mail updates from the National Oceanic and Atmospheric Administration that are forwarded to hospital management via the hospital's public information officer.

After arriving on Sunday morning, Pam goes to the administration boardroom on the first floor, where the Incident Command Center is set up. Around the boardroom table, there are briefings on the storm's status, reports from each manager on how preparations were progressing, and descriptions of any outstanding issues that need attention. A television bolted into the corner wall that faces Napoleon Avenue is tuned to the Weather Channel. People gasp when they see Hurricane Katrina's massive circular rotating image covering the entire television screen.

"Seeing that red thing coming in our direction and thinking, 'Well, this is going to happen.' It took a long time for it to sink into me that this hurricane was going to run over us. And then it did, and I still don't think I connected to what was going to happen. I wasn't scared out of my wits. I was not. I was never frightened [about] the landfall of the hurricane. I felt really comfortable that we could handle whatever it was that came our way."

As the forecast from the National Hurricane Center projects dire impact from the hurricane, Pam tells herself, "Damn, this does not sound good. And as we watched the few snippets of television on Saturday night and Sunday morning before we left home . . . with everyone on television from the local government saying it looks bad, it still did not translate to me what the experience was going to be. Obviously these people had some realization as to what we were in for."

Her husband, Roy, had stayed at the hospital with her during Hurricane Andrew, which threatened New Orleans in the early 1990s. Roy had vowed not to be there for another storm, but this time he comes. He packs an overnight bag with clothes and takes his toolbox. As soon as he arrives, he and other volunteers are assigned to help the engineering crew with final plant operation preparations. Later, he is among the employees, physicians, and volunteers who help move patients to the heliport or the emergency room (ER) ramp for evacuation. Pam says the extra manpower became essential help for the nursing department's predominately female staff.

On Sunday night, a preterm infant is born in labor and delivery. There are now 16 babies in the NICU. The NICU patients are moved to a central location in labor and delivery that has no windows. On Monday, before 5:00 a.m., windows start rattling as hurricane-force winds hammer the hospital. The women's and infants' waiting area adjacent to the newborn nursery, renovated 6 months earlier, is now filled with patient family members and visitors. As the winds intensify, the pressure change is noticed by everyone. They quickly move out of the area, away from its floor-to-ceiling windows. At that moment, ceiling tiles drop on the floor, and in the waiting area, the windows shatter. Shards of glass fall like confetti on chairs and sofas where some of the family members and visitors had been only minutes before. Fortunately, no one is injured. Rain blows in; the carpet becomes a sponge, soaked by the rain and later promoting the mold that gradually makes patterns across the walls. By mid-afternoon, Pam says they see and hear about the storm's destruction. From their sixth-floor area, the staff see the Superdome, part of its roof peeled back and exposed.

On Tuesday, August 30, the Incident Command Center moves to the fourth-floor nursing education room because the first floor is now threatened by rising water. The room has over a dozen computers, which are used by the staff to check the news and weather updates. The staff are in touch with the hospital's parent company in Dallas, which is monitoring its five New Orleans–area hospitals, and also one on the Mississippi Gulf Coast in Biloxi, 84 miles east of New Orleans. At one end of the room, a 12-inch television draws a small audience of employees and volunteers. Images are snowy, but no one complains. There is news footage of the Walmart in St. Bernard almost completely underwater, but as Pam watches, there is no word about St. Bernard Parish. Pam deals with the knowledge that her home is most likely flooded as an afterthought. It is just one more thing to deal with, but definitely not her priority right now.

"I figured that it [the aftermath of the hurricane] was very, very bad," she says. "But honestly, I just didn't even think about it."

St. Bernard Parish was home to approximately 68,000 residents. Katrina had widespread devastation from its 145-mph winds and its 25-foot storm surge. "Our homes looked like someone took a blender and churned everything. . . . It was surreal—still surreal. Tuesday night was the last time I had talked to my daughter on the phone, and she said she and her brother were really tired of being in Houston and wanted to come home. I must have realized that everything was gone on Tuesday because I said to her, 'What are you watching on TV there? We are not coming home. Home is gone.'"

At the Incident Command Center, employees are e-mailing sister hospitals (owned by their parent company) across the country for assistance in receiving all of Memorial's patients. The women's and infants' staff are advised to reach out and find a hospital that can receive their fragile babies. Everyone on the unit starts calling, using landlines and cell phones. Three of their neonatologists at Memorial Medical Center make calls as well. One physician reaches Woman's Hospital in Baton Rouge. They can take all of the babies. Destination determined, the next task is to prepare each patient for transport. Going from patient to patient, Pam takes their medical reports, gets the latest update on their status, and then begins to cohort the babies according to their medical conditions and equipment needs. Those who are ventilated are paired with the babies that are on oxygen. These patients are triaged to go out first. The rest of the patients are paired according to their needs. Each pair is laid side by side in a crib, ready for transport. For charting, the nurse practitioners write a summary sheet for each baby. These are included with the babies' most recent medical records and medications.

Communications for evacuation with the Coast Guard air resources bring more challenges. "We kept trying to tell the people who were on the other end of the phone the medical needs of our NICU patients. It became evident pretty early on in the process we could not be certain what type of medical evacuation would arrive, when it was coming, and if it would be sufficient for the needs of our patients. That's when we decided to make each baby self-contained. If the baby needed oxygen, intravenous fluids, pumps—whatever it was—each patient must have the resources needed to survive. The nurses get the oxygen tanks and fortunately, all of our equipment is well charged and ready to work on battery while taking the babies to Baton Rouge. We did not count on the rescue vehicle having any particular service that our patients would need, so we had to take it upon ourselves to supply everything that was needed."

Warming pads are placed in each crib. Some babies are equipment-dependent, in need of pumps. Those babies who are oxygen-dependent or on ventilators leave first. Pam still has the piece of paper she used to color-code the patient triage. "There was the orange group, the green group, blue group, brown group on my paper so that I knew who was actually in the bed with whom," she says.

No sooner has the staff readied their young charges when a group of employees and volunteers comes to the sixth floor—the helicopters are on their way. They need to get to the heliport now. To bring the incubators to the heliport, they pass them through what was known as the "hole," on the second floor. The "hole" is an opening that hospital engineers had made in the wall between the hospital and the garage wall that butted up against it, anticipating that one day, it would be used for an evacuation or for when the elevator to the heliport was nonfunctioning. Once through the wall, the incubators are placed, one at a time, in the back of a pick-up truck and driven up the spiraled ramp (nine floors) of the Magnolia Parking Garage. When they reach the top level, the incubator has to be carried up two flights of steep outside stairs to the heliport. However, one incubator causes a problem; its top does not clear the low garage ceiling once it is placed in the back of the truck, so they push it up the nine levels. When they reach the top of the heliport, they also discover that the ventilation mechanism is not working, maybe due to the stress encountered as they pushed it up the garage ramp. Pam counts this as a blessing.

"So there is no reason to take it. It is called a Road Runner; it weighs over 200 pounds and is designed to go in the back of an ambulance. It is not meant to go in a helicopter. The flight incubators are built of different materials, light enough to fly, and I thought, 'Oh, God, I can't think of how they are going to take off if this equipment is not meant to go into a helicopter.' But it broke. So I made the sign of the cross and said, 'Thank you, Jesus,' because I was afraid of what might have happened had they attempted to fly."

The two tiny newborns are taken out of that incubator. One is tucked inside the shirt of his nurse, the other cradled in a physician's arms. He hand-ventilates the tiny baby the entire flight to Baton Rouge, which is interrupted by a fueling stop en route. There is still twilight at 8:00 P.M. The heliport has additional lighting fashioned from flashlights the engineering staff has strung, with the use of a portable generator, around

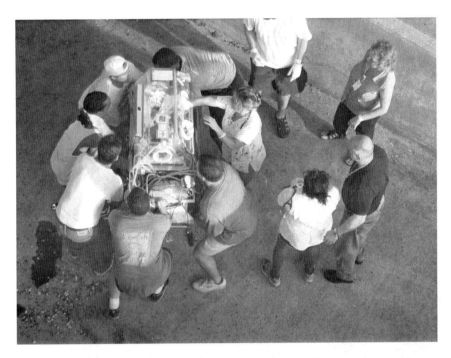

Memorial Medical Center staff and volunteers move an isolette to the hospital heliport for evacuation. All NICU patients were safely airlifted to Baton Rouge. Photo by Scarlett Welch-Nakajima.

the landing perimeter. Around 9:00 P.M., the last helicopter lifts off with the last of the NICU patients. Six hours later, the generators that had powered the NICU stop.

"One of my takeaways from this experience was that it was the right people and years of experience and the trust that we had established amongst ourselves that made it go so well. . . . After communications broke down . . . I feel that we made good decisions and I think that came from experience. The people who I had worked with for so long really trusted what I had to say, and they were self-directed. I trusted them to carry out the task and I didn't try to micromanage. That allowed me to move on to the next task. I really think that the combination of the trust and the experience in the people who were there really made a huge difference. People had their momentary meltdowns, myself included, but nobody became nonfunctional."

The parents of the NICU babies leave by boat during the next day and reach family members, who later meet them in Baton Rouge, reunited with their babies. The NICU cleared of patients, the staff now has to focus on evacuating the five newborns in the well-baby nursery. They manage to get all the babies and their mothers out together by boat to the Jefferson Parish line. From there, an ambulance takes the mothers and babies to Baton Rouge. "Still it had not sunk in that we were all going to be leaving and never coming back," Pam recalls.

The women's and infants' staff join other employees, who are on the lower floors with patients who have been relocated to the main lobby and the ER ramp. The patients are laid out on mattresses and cots on the floor. They are continuously fanned by nurses, volunteers, and even children of employees. A couple of them, exhausted from the heat, do not feel they could do even that task. Their colleagues take their place. By the evening of Wednesday, August 31, all of the women's and infants' services staff have moved from the various units in the maternal–child area on the sixth floor into the NICU, also located on the sixth floor. It also houses an assortment of pets, including a Great Dane, a hedgehog, cats, and even a squirrel. The broken windows in the waiting area allow the flow of cooler air, but the heat hangs in the air. Tiled flooring offers a cool surface on which to sleep. Outside the double glass doors that lead to the nursery and the NICU, Roy and George (husband of one of Pam's nurses) guard the one door that opens at the front of the nursery. They also escort the nurses to their assignments in others areas of the hospital because the nursing staff is scared to walk through the dark hospital.

"That night, I was walking through the second floor, and all of a sudden [I see] these guys in a full costume from hat to boots and the big guns—oh, the cavalry is here." The "cavalry" was the New Orleans Police Department SWAT team. They were responding to a distress call they received from someone at the hospital. They had arrived at the ER ramp, where Denise Danna, chief nursing officer, and a few of her colleagues were trying to find a cool evening breeze. "We heard the sound of guns cocked and someone said, 'Turn off those flashlights.' They said they got a call . . . there was a shooting going on in the hospital. And they went through the hospital, but they wouldn't stay. They said their job was to come in and make sure there wasn't anything going on and they left," Denise explains to Pam, 3 years after the event. But at the time, Pam knew no different and went back to tell her staff everything was under control and that the army had arrived. Her news was greeted with cheers. Later that night, the husband of the assistant head nurse shows the symptoms of a heart attack. They place him on a heart monitor and give him oxygen and medication.

"I had a couple of people ask me, 'Are we going to die?' I said, 'No, we are not going to die.' That was the answer. In the meantime, I was thinking, 'I don't know . . .' What freaked me out was seeing everything on fire. When I looked out and saw everything burning around us, I thought, 'That is not the way I want to go. What are we going to do if we catch on fire?' That was one of my biggest worries."

Pam now looks at emergency preparedness drills with a new post-storm perspective. "Don't ever think that this can't happen to you. You are going to read this and it's going to sound like we created this scenario, but this really happened. What would you do?"

On the sixth floor, Pam says she and the staff were isolated from communications and activities in other areas of the hospital. She knew her staff, as nurses, were prepared to go in as part of Team A, but her concerns were now also about their spouses and children. "My poor husband is helping transfer a patient in a wheelchair up the stairs. . . . The lady kept taking her hospital gown and wiped his face telling him, 'Thank you for saving my life, thank you, honey, for saving my life.' There was another lady they'd fan and fan and fan. She was senile, and every now and then she'd have some lucidity. She was cracking Roy up telling him all kinds of stuff. He spent some time fanning her, and next thing she is up on the heliport and he said, 'I think she is dead.' Then there was the guy that came in who had been stabbed. And the 90-year-old man who kept them in stitches the whole time telling stories and jokes. Roy and another volunteer put both of them in the same helicopter."

Come Thursday, September 1, the entire hospital is in full evacuation mode. Pam says people were evacuated from the first floor of the Clara Wing on boats and helicopters. She describes the scene "like someone had stepped on an ant pile." On the stairs, Pam encounters a woman and her husband, who has had recent heart surgery. As a team of employees and volunteers move the patient up the stairs to the heliport, his wife becomes frantic, asking Pam what she is going to do with her bags. Pam tells her she can only take one bag. This upsets the woman. Pam tells the others to keep moving and she will stay with the woman and assist her up the stairs. Visibly shaken, the woman turns to Pam and shows her two cats inside the bag.

"She asks, 'What am I going to do with my cats?' Fortunately, I saw one of my colleague's husbands, who I knew was a gentle soul. I told her the animal control people have been called and they are coming as soon as the hospital has been vacated to get all of the animals. So I am going to take your cats to a place where the animal control people can pick them up. And Howard passed by, and I said, 'Howard, would you please take these two cats for me?' Howard took the cats, and the lady and I went up the steps, and when we got to the top we couldn't find her husband. He had been evacuated."

Pam begins to feel that the 5 days is taking a toll on her. She feels that her body is going into total shutdown. She looks at her colleagues, and they are exhausted from the unrelenting oppressive heat and manual labor. Around 3:30 P.M. on Thursday, Pam and a few of her colleagues stand on the hospital ER ramp watching boats load their passengers. An administrator turns to her group and tells them to go. So with two of her colleagues, a physician, and two cats, they leave. "I think it was just a matter of timing," Pam sighs. "We had been up and down the hospital steps the whole time and there was this collection of us on the emergency room ramp and we were told 'get your party and get out of here on this boat.'"

From the hospital, the boat heads along Napoleon Avenue, south toward the Mississippi River. Slowly the boat passes submerged cars, some with water past their roofs. Debris of trash, wood, and clothing floats on top of the water. The water is streaked with an oily stain that shimmers in the hot sun. One block before reaching St. Charles Avenue, about a half mile from Memorial Medical Center, the passengers get out of the boat and step into a foot of water. They walk past Pascal Manale's Restaurant and reach St. Charles Avenue. They look for the buses that they were told would take them to a triage area. There are cars and the Audubon Zoo mobile, but no buses. A long line of people snakes along the Napoleon Avenue neutral ground where the St. Charles streetcars traveled. Pam sees some hospital employees pooling their cash to pay the driver of a truck to take them to Baton Rouge. An ambulance drives up with one of the hospital physicians. They load a handful of the nurses and leave. As Pam stands in line with her colleagues, officers from the New Orleans Police Department approach them. With them is an elderly woman.

"She looked 90—Miss Kitty. They found Miss Kitty wandering on the street and said, 'You're from the hospital so can you please take care of Miss Kitty?' Miss Kitty had a cigarette and a dollar bill, and at some point in time, we wrote her name and put it in her pocket. We waited and waited and waited to get to the interstate." A few hours passed, and Pam's group hitches a ride in a van. Sitting inside on the van floor, no one has any idea about their destination. When the van stops, they get out at the Causeway and Interstate 10 cloverleaf. This was an evacuation staging area. Pam says, "It was a scene out of like the end of the world."

There are throngs of people of all ages. Some look dazed. Others sit on blankets or suitcases. Children are crying. The stench of human waste and rotting food is hard to avoid.

"Of course, I am thinking, 'It can't be any worse than what it was at the hospital,'" says Pam. "We asked, 'Where do we sign in?' and they laugh at us. So we start walking around trying to figure out what is going on. There were some people from Memorial. There was a constant, continuous line of people, a deep line waiting for buses to come, and some people did get on a bus while we were there. There was no order. Nobody was in charge. Nobody!

"Then we said, 'We cannot keep Miss Kitty. There is no way we can do this.' There was a medical station out on the interstate, and we gave Miss Kitty over to them. We wandered around the area and then decided we were going to walk away to safety. We climbed a fence, got on the service road, and we started walking toward Cleary Avenue. When we left, there was a medical tent with an ambulance there."

It is near sundown. Pam and her group still have not been able to find anyone who can tell them who is in charge of the evacuee site by the interstate. They overhear that Jefferson Parish deputies are told shoot to kill suspect looters and other vagrants. As darkness descends, they decide to turn around and return to the cloverleaf on the interstate, after hearing the orders that were given to the deputies. When they get to the site, they find that the medical personnel who had been working there were packing up to leave. "They [the medical personnel] told us first of all, 'We are not safe, we have nobody to keep us safe here and we don't have any more supplies that we need so we are just getting out of here.' They left. As we are walking back by the concrete barriers . . . there were body bags stacked in between the concrete road barriers. . . . There was nobody in charge. You couldn't talk to the state police, you couldn't talk to the National Guard," she says.

A convoy of the National Guard drives by the area. Pam says it is like a Mardi Gras parade of trucks, with the soldiers throwing meals ready to eat (MREs) and cots into the crowd. By now, there are 40 people from Memorial Medical Center in Pam's group. They manage to get a few cots and MREs and leave the zone where the buses are supposed to arrive. Pam picks up a plastic mattress on the ground. The area smells like human waste. From their new vantage point, they watch as more hospital workers from other facilities are dropped off at the cloverleaf.

Pam's group rests on the ground. Through the night, the group from Memorial Medical Center tries to be as low key as possible. Then, about

5:30 A.M., a civil defense volunteer from LaPlace walks up toward the entire crowd. He approaches the area where Pam and her colleagues are gathered and tells them quietly that if they can walk slowly and quietly past the crowd, he has a truck and will take them to LaPlace. They follow him. But as they reach the truck, people from the crowd surge toward the truck. Pam looks at one of the elderly parents in her group. "I said, 'I can't do this. I want the elderly people to get on the truck first.' So we let the others get on the truck and they take off with the first go-round. At this time, we are well past the crowd.

"Refrigerator trucks are all lined up on the interstate waiting for the dead people. When I look at who has come with us, I realize we left behind Miss Elaine, an employee who is 72, from Memorial's postpartum unit. Not everybody came! And it totally overwhelms me. I wanted to go back to get her. They said, 'You cannot go back into that crowd.' 'But we came with these people here, we cannot leave them here.'" She shrugs. "I didn't get my wish, which would have been to go back. I was so overwhelmed for so long that we left Miss Elaine behind. To this day, that is one of the things that makes me upset if I really think about it because we had taken care of each other this far, for us to have left some of our people behind. . . . I think eventually they got out somehow, but I don't know exactly what happened to her. She was 72 and she had her daughter, her little dog, and she was still in her uniform looking meticulous like she always did. To this day, I don't know if I will ever reconcile myself with that."

The sun slowly rises and the group consensus is that the rescuer is not returning. But he does. Fourteen of them get into the truck. There is only room for three in the front cabin. The others climb onto the flatbed. One girl lies across the tailgate, while the others hold on to each other and to her, to keep her from falling off as the driver speeds at 50 mph across the Bonnet Carre Spillway to LaPlace.

"All I could do is put my head down, and I said the rosary the whole time." Safe in LaPlace, they arrive at a government center. A volunteer at the center knows where Roy's cousin lives and drives them to his home. He is cutting his lawn when they pull up in his driveway. Four years later, Pam says post-traumatic stress has had an effect on her children, who, for 3 days, thought their parents were dead. Her daughter becomes upset and assumes the worst if she cannot reach a family member. Her son graduated in May 2006. No family member of hers, on both sides of the family, had a home—not one.

"To this day, memories of the hospital experience are in a box," she says. "A big box of something that sits on the shelf. When I got the DVD that one of the nurses made of the evacuation, I was in Baton Rouge. I can remember sitting in the closet and I cried till my nightgown was saturated. I cried and I cried and I cried. The couple of times that I watched it were very emotional. After we left the hospital, there was so much to do personally that I could not connect to what had happened there.

"And lately, I have been dreaming about the hospital a lot. I dream that I am back there. In one of the dreams, I was back on the sixth floor. I remember Jo, in particular, was working, Dana was working, and I was there, but I couldn't participate. I couldn't be part of the work. And I have been dreaming a lot about being a bedside nurse again. It comes and goes."

She feels that employees did not have the opportunity for closure. She understands why the hospital was closed. "We needed help. We needed closure. We had no closure, no ability to go back to our place."

It matters to her that others understand and appreciate the breadth and depth of Hurricane Katrina's impact. "Anything can happen to anybody at any point in time, and you owe it to yourself and your family— the people to whom you are accountable—to be ready for what can possibly happen. I think it's a testimony to what you can do when you are put in the position of having to do superhuman feats. And you know, people ask me, 'Would you do it again?' And my answer to that is, 'Well, you know, I am not feeling like I need to sign up to go to a hospital again to seek out that experience,' but if I was in a hospital and knowing the consequences, both emotional and physical . . . all of the consequences that came after, I'm a nurse, and that's what my role is—take care of people . . . and if I couldn't find myself able emotionally or physically, [if] I didn't think I had the stamina to do it, then probably the hospital isn't the place for me to be."

In December 2006, Pam's family moves back into her rebuilt home, located behind historic Jackson Barracks in St. Bernard Parish. She considers herself fortunate that her raised house took on only 3 feet of water. The homecoming was good, yet bittersweet. It was almost a repeat of 1965, when Hurricane Betsy ravaged St. Bernard Parish and left Pam and her family stranded on the roof of their house. But the neighborhood rebuilt then. Now, 40 years later, everyone in her family had lost their homes—parents, mother-in-law, her husband's siblings, cousins.

Her brother-in-law's grandmother died at St. Rita's Nursing Home. No one in her family returned to St. Bernard Parish. Her husband's uncle and one cousin were the only ones who decided to rebuild. "I will never forget the Monday my parents met up with us in Baton Rouge," she offers. "All they had were their luggage, a couple of shopping bags, and a Rubbermaid bin. That was what was left of their life. I still get pretty overwhelmed thinking that good people could live for 70 years and be reduced to a Rubbermaid bin."

"What's interesting about people who are from St. Bernard is that those of us who live in St. Bernard don't feel like we're home. Those of us who are displaced don't feel like they're home. So nobody I feel has made a whole heck of a lot of progress in moving on. You know, sometimes we just go drive around. Like we drove to my mom's driveway and looked at her slab the other day. We took pictures. Roy and I drove around one day when they first started the house demolitions. We took stupid pictures like sitting in my brother's backyard on the portion of his deck that was left, and all this debris all over the place. We took a picture in a boat on his front lawn. It was difficult to go back. It's sad. It's just really, really sad. I went to Walgreens last night and realized everything is gone. It is disorientating, even when you live out there."

Pam's return to the clinical setting is brief. She tries both clinical and nonclinical settings, but they lack the structure, responsibilities, and respect that she expects the job to offer from managers and administrators. She encounters resentment from nurses when she challenges them on ways to do some tasks. "I never felt comfortable because I've never found the same degree of support, professionalism, just everything that we had [at Memorial] there makes it real difficult to go out and try to integrate. Were we an anomaly? I think now that maybe we were.

"I was so lucky to have the years of service at Memorial. The people I met, both patients and coworkers, have so shaped my life. I just need to figure out how to channel that experience into my new life in order to make a difference again. I don't know how it happened, but so many of us who thought alike and worked alike assembled in one place."

She credits an epiphany that prompted her to start working on a master's degree in nursing, explaining, "If I am not going to be part of the problem, I need to be part of the solution. What am I going to do? I have no idea, but I am here. And I daily just try to frame up my expectations to be reasonable."

She has coauthored two articles about the evacuation and emergency preparedness. Another paper has been accepted for presentation

at the September 2009 conference of the National Association of Neonatal Nurses. "We have been able to tell our story in the national forum
and that was also so surreal to me.

"My other goal is, nobody should ever have to do this again. No nurse,
no patient, no one, should ever have to suffer like all the staff did."

Jarrett Fuselier

*We are going to ride this out. We are going to do what we need to
do, and when it is time to go, we are gonna go. We decided that's
just how it's going to be.*

Jarrett Fuselier, RN, BSN, MBA, earned a bachelor's degree in nursing
from LSUHSC in 2001 and a master's degree in business administration
with a concentration in health care management from the University
of New Orleans (UNO) in 2004. He is currently employed at a medical
center on the West Bank as the unit director of ICU/cardiology and the
cath lab.

Saturday is a day of celebration for Jarrett and his family. It is his daughter's first birthday. He and his wife are getting ready for the party at their
Luling home in St. Charles Parish, a 30-minute drive due west of New
Orleans. The watermelon was chilled, hot dogs and chili were ready—but
plans soon changed. The storm is steering toward New Orleans. His wife
and daughter leave for Lafayette, Louisiana. The house was still.

A staff nurse in the surgical ICU at Memorial Medical Center, Jarrett is on the hospital's Team A, which reports to work for storms and any
other major emergency. He has worked every storm, with the exception
of one. Now there is a mass churning in the Gulf of Mexico. He expects
it to blow through and that he'll be home the following afternoon. On
Sunday, August 28, he awakens around 2:00 A.M. and turns on the television. "I saw that big old buzz saw of 175-mph winds," says Jarrett. "When
I got ready to go to work, I called my dad, who worked for Entergy.
I said, 'Hey man, are you going to able to get a helicopter to come pick
me up at work if we're flooded?' He said, 'Whatever, just go to work.'
I said, 'OK, I will call you when I am on my way home.'"

Although he is scheduled to work Monday, he goes to the hospital
Sunday morning around 10 A.M. to help with prep work and assess inventories of supplies and linens. He brings with him a change of clothes
and the birthday fare that will become supper for coworkers and physicians later that night. The ICU is located in the New Orleans Surgery

and Heart Institute. Employees call it NOSHI. The four-story building was for the former Eye, Ear, Nose, and Throat Hospital. In 2001, when Jarrett was hired, NOSHI had been converted to support surgical and cardiac services. On the third floor are 13 operating rooms and three cath labs. The 20-bed surgical ICU (SICU) is on the second floor. The patient rooms face a windowed wall that fronts Napoleon Avenue. The staff board up some of the windows. An enclosed covered walkway on the second floor connects the building to the main hospital.

On the morning of Monday, August 29, the SICU staff move their patients to the hospital's eighth floor—the former surgery floor before its 2001 move across the street. By Monday evening, Jarrett says, "We knew that things weren't going to be normal. We weren't going to be going home the next day." On Tuesday, the water starts rising along the streets. "One of our nurses whose home was near the lakefront campus of the University of New Orleans hears from her husband. The water is rising and he is leaving their home in search of higher ground. He ended up on one of the overpasses the last time we heard," says Jarrett. "The water was coming from the lake. We knew it wasn't going to be a good thing. The water wasn't going to go away quickly. We didn't know all of the chaos going around in the city."

That morning, Jarrett positions himself with his colleagues on the heliport of the hospital. From that vantage point, they can see the waters that surrounded the hospital's four-city-block campus. The neighborhood is a lake that stretches toward downtown. When air traffic slows, they take a break. An intermittent cool breeze gives respite from the August heat. They take turns working at the ER ramp, where they help to load evacuating patients and family members on boats. They relieve fellow employees and volunteers, who are fanning patients with sheets of cardboard. He tries to sleep an hour or two each night.

Dietary services are relocated from the basement to the fourth floor of the hospital before the flooding claims the cafeteria as well as laundry, computer services, and engineering. Using hot plates, breakfast is grits, scrambled eggs, and sausage, served in a Styrofoam cup, for everyone in the hospital. "Almost seems like we got hot meals longer than we should have, but I never got hungry," recalls Jarrett. "[It] wasn't much, but it was nice to actually get a little."

His group of ICU nurses gets facility updates. Periodically, an administrator enlists them for assignments in other areas of the hospital. From the beginning, the task of moving the patients up the flights of

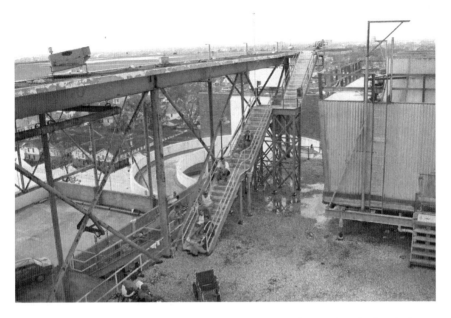

Memorial Medical Center staff and volunteers wait with patients below the hospital heliport for the next helicopter. Photo by Sandra E. Cordray.

stairs is physically daunting. The carved hole in the garage wall, used to expedite patient evacuation, is a lifesaver, proclaims Jarrett. Patients are passed through the four-by-four opening directly to the garage, where they are placed on the back of a truck and driven to the top level of the ninth floor, just below the heliport.

"This always gets me: The state people said we were trying to make people 'do not resuscitate' [DNR] and leave them there, but one of my patients, a DNR . . . we brought him up to the helipad and transported him out because we were triaging them out that morning. Getting the sickest patients out first. He was one of the first patients to go." By Wednesday, communications become sporadic. There are reports of civil disorder in the city. However, Jarrett is oblivious to that. Power is out, and there seems to be an unending flow of work to be done. Blackness settles over the city as night comes. The hospital stairwells are lit by a trail of flashlights. Communication is by word of mouth, which filters down the human chain assembled to carry each patient. Some are lifted in wheelchairs. Others are wrapped in bedsheets or placed on spine boards. At nightfall, the air evacuation ceases, to resume the following morning.

"We'd rest a little bit at night, but we would go around and fan the patients, a few comforting things we could do for them at that point. And we just stayed busy. We didn't want to sit down and do nothing. . . . The whole time I was never really worried. . . . I had my group of coworkers and friends who were going to ride this out. We are going to do what we need to do, and when it is time to go, we are going to go. We decided that's just how it's going to be." As they wait with patients underneath the heliport, the staff get their patients ready and await a signal from the helicopter pilot one level above them. When they get the go-ahead they can mobilize and take the metal stairs to the landing pad. One helicopter crew drops off a satellite phone that does not work.

On Wednesday, two physicians leave the hospital in search of dry land. Boats from the Wildlife and Fisheries Department begin arriving. Recalls Jarrett, shaking his head, "We thought we were dropping the patients and staff off somewhere better, but that was not what happened. You do the best thing you can at the time."

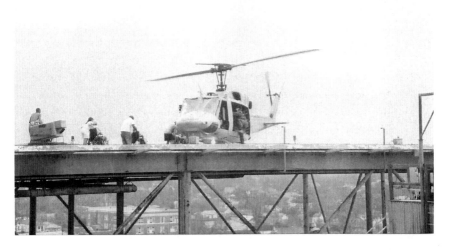

Patients are wheeled to a waiting helicopter on the Memorial Medical Center heliport. Photo by Scarlett Welch-Nakajima.

He says he knew it was bad the day when Air Force One flew over as they sat near the helipad with their patients. "When you see the whole city full of water, it is not a good thing." Despite the challenges, he says the staff worked well together. "We couldn't have everybody concentrated on patient care, but everybody was focused on the patients. Everybody came to kind of own an area, whether it was the people moving the patients; those taking care of the ones in the garage, on the second floor or the [emergency room]. Everybody did their best, whether it was pointing the fan on the patient with our little fan brigades we had in the middle of the night. Everybody understood that it was bad. People stayed relatively calm. It was kind of surprising . . . the staff you'd expect to be OK, but when you have the 2,000 others . . ."

Mid-morning on Thursday, September 1, a physician motions to Jarrett and three of his comrades. They need workers to assist those who are being dropped off by the boats. They take the next boat out to where the water levels off, a half block shy of the intersection of St. Charles Avenue and Napoleon Avenue. They roll a stretcher through the waters to the idling boats and help the less ambulatory people disembark. When they arrive, there is a small crowd gathering at the corner.

"We said, 'Look, we need this area, can you clear out?' They listened, for some weird reason." Tarps are spread out and water offered to the new arrivals. A few policemen stand nearby. "Some guy from the levee board actually showed up early that morning. He was looking for a patient. Somehow we hooked up with him early and kept in touch with him all day to try and secure a ride out," says Jarrett.

When the first group from Memorial arrives, there are no buses. A small group of ambulances from Houston is parked at the intersection. They take one of the staff physicians and three employees. Jarrett's group later gets word that the ambulances are not returning "because they heard they weren't going to get paid. That wasn't nice of them. Then there was this other guy—Pace. He had eight ambulances . . . just drove down with his ambulances from north Louisiana. He came down; had his Suburban . . . helped us load them up . . . they were taking the patients away. They were coming back. We kept loading them up and taking them out. Patients, employees, everybody was going." The steady exit of people is comprised mainly of employees, family members, and pets. Throughout the day, the boats keep coming to deposit their cargo. Some passengers stay near the tarped area. Others cross the street to wait for a bus or whatever vehicle that will take passengers. Residents from the neighborhood mill about. Jarrett says the people who had come from the hospital were relatively calm. "Nobody hysterical, nobody upset."

The Copeland's Restaurant on one corner has been raided. Smiles Jarrett, "Somebody was nice enough to take all of the furniture out of Copeland's and set it out there, so we set the chairs up. Everybody was relatively comfortable." The Walgreens on the corner diagonal to the restaurant has a steady flow of traffic through the looted store. "Police were saying, 'You need something, go into Walgreens,'" says Jarrett. Someone tried to break into a car. Two National Guard soldiers patrol the area, holding their guns near their shoulders. "When we saw the guys with the guns walking through the streets, we realized it was bad. Looked like it was a different country."

Around 5:00 P.M., the police announce that they are shutting down the activity because of safety concerns. The police have limited communications with each other. We tried to see if they could clear some way for the ambulances when they were getting out, and they just weren't able to communicate with anybody to get them through," says Jarrett. Now only a handful of people are at the intersection at St. Charles and Napoleon. The last group of hospital employees has boarded a bus. It has been nearly 7 hours that Jarrett and his friends have been helping to clear the area. The guy, Pace, says he is staying in LaPlace. He offers to take them with him and drop them off at Jarrett's house, or at the house of Jarrett's friend and fellow nurse.

And then Jarrett hears someone shout his name. He turns. It is his father-in-law, a fire chief in St. Charles Parish. He has been looking for Jarrett all day.

"Earlier in the day, I met this Japanese reporter who couldn't understand English. We had a communication problem, and I ended up using his phone. . . . I talked with my family once before we left that morning, told them we were getting out. I said, 'You'll find me on St. Charles or walking to Harahan along River Road. Come pick me up. This is where we are going to be. If not, we'll manage.'"

His father-in-law had been driving along the Mississippi River levee looking for him and was as close as the river side of St. Charles Avenue, but they could not see each other—a block away, they had missed each other. He retraces his route and stops at a hospital in Jefferson that is not flooded. Someone tells him to look for Jarrett back at St. Charles and Napoleon avenues. It is almost 6:00 P.M. Jarrett and his coworkers finally have a ride out. He joins his family in Lafayette. After a few minutes of watching the news coverage, it is clear to Jarrett how bad the situation had been for the city.

Communication flow, he says, is just as critical today as it was after Hurricane Katrina. "Keep those lines of communication clear as possible. Everything was pretty good for how bad it was. Don't know if it is just nurses, but everybody pretty much comes together, does what they need to do, what they need to get done. Not everybody is going to do everything, but everybody is going to fill that void, and people appreciate what little communication they get—whatever information. And they want to feel that it is genuine information and you are not just telling them that just to pacify them. Most of the information we had going out was as good information as we knew at that point, and I think that's what helped."

The October after Hurricane Katrina, Jarrett returns to nursing. Today, he is director of ICU and the cath lab at a facility on the West Bank of New Orleans, where he saw firsthand patient evacuation for Hurricane Gustav. It was clear that evacuation protocols were impacted by the Katrina experiences.

Jarrett was pushing for evacuation of his patients in the ICU. "Administration said, 'The patients can be evacuated in the morning.' I said, 'We need to do it now.' I woke up at four in the morning and said, 'Why haven't we moved anybody yet?' I called the transfer center of the hospital, and they said we had time. I said, 'Yeah, we have time, but we need to get them moving now.' And they did. We started moving people. . . . We didn't know what could happen the first time, but now that we knew what could happen, try to prevent that from happening. Staff complained it was chaotic when we were moving patients; coming too fast. Next time, it will be a little better."

Jo Lincks

> *[I] could not accept that being an American that I would be in this situation.*

Jo Lincks, RN, is a native of New Orleans. Jo graduated from LSU School of Nursing with a bachelor of science degree in 1974. For most of her career, she has been a nurse in the NICU and well-baby nursery areas. She is currently employed at a New Orleans–area hospital as a staff nurse in the well-baby nursery.

Jo admits that she came to work with no trepidation about the hurricane. "My intuition must have been totally shut off. . . . I am the person that brings boxes of food because I can't stand the thought of not having food. And this time I brought hardly anything. I thought that we would be going home in a couple of days. I brought my grandson, my daughter-in-law, her mother from Brazil, and her friend who doesn't speak English. But they got out"—her intuition was working—"my daughter-in-law." When her son, a photographer for a local television station, calls to tell her that they are relocating their operation to Baton Rouge, she realizes that her family members need to leave the hospital that Sunday night. "Thank God. If I had to go through it with them, I would have had more anger," she says.

She spends most of her time on the sixth floor, in the well-baby nursery or in labor and delivery. When she leaves the area, it is to help fan patients and, later, to push wheelchairs up the garage ramp that leads to the heliport, where patients are airlifted by the military, Coast Guard, and private helicopters.

On Monday, she sleeps in labor and delivery, where the newborns have been moved because of concerns about the nursery windows breaking from the anticipated high winds. Around 4:30 A.M., electricity goes out and emergency generator power kicks in. The storm passes, and Jo begins her 7:00 A.M. to 3:00 P.M. shift. "Until the water started rising, we were relieved that we had weathered the storm," she says. "Tuesday, people started getting nervous when the water started coming up. Some parents were able to communicate with people on the outside. One family actually left. They talked with someone who knew a route to use to get out before the water would get high enough. They left and they did OK. That night people were getting tired and scared."

During the storm, Jo says she took on the role of spiritual director in the nursery. "I was a confidante—people talked," she says. "I was always supportive, mostly because of my own belief. I genuinely believed, and I would tell them, look at the people who are here. These are the people who are supposed to be here. Look at how we worked like a well-oiled machine."

She applauds the leadership of her director, Pam. "I watched. Everything she had ever done in her career she utilized in getting everything done. The transport. She knew it. She was able to pull all that knowledge about what to fit where. And the respect that she had garnered from all of us that we listened to her. Whatever she said do, we did. She had such a relationship with the NICU nurses she didn't have to tell them. They knew.

"And Danielle, professional throughout. Totally professional. There is nothing any of us wouldn't have done for either of those women. The power of a good manager. Again, I took for granted at Baptist Hospital, and I haven't found what I had there again. I haven't seen it anywhere. I am sure it exists in the United States, but probably not New Orleans right now."

By Wednesday, all NICU and well-baby nursery babies have been successfully evacuated from the hospital. While she is fanning patients who have been gathered in the second-floor atrium, a colleague finds Jo. It is time to go. Jo is elated by the news, but the feeling is short-lived. It is a false start. She returns to the atrium to resume her work.

When speaking about her fellow nurses, she calls them professionals who never considered abandoning their patients. "That wasn't ever even a thought. I think people, in the back of their minds, thought some one was coming—somebody was going to come. But you could tell [those] people who were not sure their families were safe because some of the nurses had left their children at home. There was some real agony, some angst."

She recalls Wednesday evening as "a hard night." If one of the nurses in her unit has an assignment in another area of the hospital, she is escorted by one of the nurses' husbands, who are part of the volunteer corps. The staff chain the entry doors to their unit. Two men stand guard at their entrance because of reports of outsiders trying to loot hospitals in search of narcotics. Jo records her thoughts in her journal:

Journal Entry: August 31, 2005

That night we took one-hour-long shifts helping out with patients on 2nd floor and older patients in 1st floor lobby. We all slept in NICU/NBN area. (Safety in numbers) Roy (St. Roy) bolted up the place with duct tape and wood. He escorted each nurse, hourly, to her assignment.

That night—Cindy got weak and saw stars.

Mike had an IV started and oxygen

Erin may also have required IV fluids.

I sat in the lounge and chatted with three young girls and Cindy and a few others.

By Thursday, some of them are succumbing to the 4 days of physical stress and heat. People are getting ill. The husband of one nurse is placed on a heart monitor. A young girl receives intravenous fluids for dehydration. Feeling abandoned, some people believe they are in mortal danger. Jo is steadfast that rescuers are on their way with help. "I knew they were coming to save us. I heard the ship was coming with the sailors. That is where I wanted to go. And I believed all those things happening and in my mind, because I am an American citizen, I know about the military and what they have available to them. I always knew they were coming. . . . I think that was the biggest disappointment.

Even when she and her colleagues are deposited at a staging area at the Interstate 10 and Causeway intersection in nearby Jefferson Parish, she has faith. But by now, it is evident that all of them are reaching their physical limitations. Thousands of evacuees, from infants to the elderly, mingle in clusters. The August heat and humidity are a taxing combination. Jo takes in the sight and thinks to herself that among this sea of humanity could have been one of her family members had they not left the city before the storm came. "That was probably the hardest thing for my psyche," she says. Chartered buses from various states are parked in a line along the shoulder of the westbound interstate. Metal barricades flank their sides, and people stand in line waiting their turn to board. A half dozen parked school buses and ambulances face eastward toward New Orleans. Helicopters periodically land to deposit more evacuees. License plates on the waiting vehicles read "Texas," "Florida," "Missouri," and other states.

When a bus joins the end of this row, a crowd surges toward it. People jostle to be first in line. They are desperate to board in the hope of being whisked away—away from the garbage spread like confetti across the landscape, away from the flattened cardboard boxes being used as pallets. They want to leave the stench and the human suffering. And then the buses stop coming. But Jo feels safe and confident surrounded by her colleagues and their family members. They share MREs, which have been tossed to the crowd from a passing National Guard truck. Even a cot offers ample room for two of them to share. A physician in their group has her cat in tow. Jo calls her "wild, curses like a sailor. She calls me Mary Poppins." Jo adds that she kept the e-mail address from that physician. It is stored with her journal and other notes.

Journal Entry: September 1, 2005, about 1:30 P.M.

We boated to St. Charles and Napoleon (waded part of the way) and waited in line for a ride to wherever. Policeman gave us 84y/o "Miss Kitty," a woman he found wandering alone down St. Charles Ave.

An ambulance with Baptist people stopped and called for Marirose to join them—but she would not leave her cat . . . so Lynn and Cindy went with them. We got into a white van with a family. They said they had spent the night in the McFarland Building—they even had hospital bracelets.

We arrived at I-10 and causeway (HELL) at about 1400–1430. We gave "Miss Kitty" to the State Police. We saw Debbie. She was in line to be the nurse for an old people bus.

A doctor was trying to get a news crew to drive us somewhere. . . . Debbie said that we might all be able to get on a bus as medical people. I said this out loud to Pam and people in the crowd heard me and made threatening remarks.

We decided to try to walk to home of the older couple's son. Pam, Roy, me, and a physician and another nurse set out on foot. It started getting dark and no one was on the street, so we decided to return (to HELL). When we arrived (after seeing body bags on the Highway; we noticed that the medical people from Texas were gone) we saw Debbie and all the medical people from Baptist had banded together for safety—under the overpass—away from the HELL people.

Debbie continuously reminded the State Police and National Guard that we were medical people, we felt unsafe, we've been working for days without sleep—we needed to be evacuated.

We ate our MRE's and slept on the ground, alternating with our 2 cots.

"I have such an admiration for all of the people I was with that I felt that we would always make the right decisions," she says. When they do leave, Jo calls their escape "miraculous." A man with a truck has come from LaPlace to help. But the task is challenging because many in this restless crowd have been at the interstate for 2 days. Two soldiers approach the Memorial group and quietly direct them where to rendezvous with this Good Samaritan. Jo says there is no formal decision making about who would leave. A group of them get up and walk to the rendezvous point. The first group leaves. No one in the crowd seems to notice their departure. The others wait in the darkness.

"Every time we'd see lights coming, we'd think it was him and it wasn't, so we already had a plan. We were going to walk to LaPlace," says Jo. "And if the guy hadn't come back I felt that we could walk to Baton Rouge or LaPlace. My life depended on it. It was all of those little things I think that kept me going. There were periods of concern. There were moments . . . I am proud of everybody who was there and how they handled it. I never saw anybody lose it. Periods of sadness perhaps, but nobody going nuts, hysterical, or anything like that.

"I didn't think we would get out that night—this miraculous guy, I have his name written, too. He and his brother were doing rescue, and he was going to drive one more time to LaPlace, come back to get us, and then he and his brother were going to get a boat the next morning and go do what they could do to help others. Those people are—how do people get like that? I don't know if I would have done that. As a layperson, me, I would have saved my family and been gone. It was a dream the way things worked out." Jo and her comrades wedge themselves onto the truck bed. She holds on to the hand of a nurse sitting on the edge of the open truck gate, fearful the woman will fall from the truck as it speeds away from the staging area.

Safe in LaPlace, Jo breaks down when she is given a phone to call her brother. She is unable to dial the number and hands the phone to someone, who makes the call. Her brother comes and takes her to Plaucheville, Louisiana, where she stays briefly with her sister-in-law's family. When electricity is restored at her brother's home in Hammond, she stays with his family until residents are allowed to return to her neighborhood. She believes what her son witnessed as he covered the storm and its aftermath through his camera lens has impacted him. "At one point he did not know if I was alive. I think the experience has some-how changed his paradigm of what life is." She will work in a hospital for another storm. "I don't have any problems with that. I feel that the system has changed. I don't think that could happen again . . . but, if so, the whole world will have its eyes on it."

On December 19, 2005, over 3 months after the storm, she re-turns to work at a hospital near her home on the West Bank. She ex-periences culture shock there, and she misses her Memorial family. In 2007, she accepts a job in the well-baby nursery at another New Or-leans hospital. To this day, she keeps in close contact with her former colleagues via a Web site that one of them created shortly after the storm. It has been Jo's lifeline to the women who became interwoven with her personal and social world during her 18 years at the hospital. They have a history, a bond. They shared with each other baby show-ers, birthdays, children's graduations. They remain connected despite the closure of the hospital where many of them had worked together for almost 2 decades.

She wants others to know how well the nurses performed in an un-imaginable situation and that a disaster of similar magnitude to Hur-ricane Katrina can happen. "I want them to know how well the nurses performed and I'd like them know there were some real heroes there.

"We weathered the storm like we always did. What we weren't able to do was function in an impossible situation," she offers. "People who were supposed to do their part didn't do their part and in spite of that . . . I am grateful to people like the man with the truck who got us out. . . . Those people from the Wildlife and Fisheries, wherever they came from, other people with their boats who came to save us. I think that's another thing that changed my outlook, I honestly believed in life that there is honor among thieves; that, in a crisis, there would be an honor among thieves. The fact that the people from wherever they were from, that there was no honor, that they genuinely were threatening us. We did watch them loot and stuff like that. That surprised me. And later, on the TV, seeing police looting . . . I didn't think people would get [to] that level. I thought that in a universal crisis even that element would perform well, would come to the rescue of basic humanity. . . . That was a big lesson for me."

Cheryl Barré

One of the young guys said, "Don't talk, ma'am. Look straight ahead. They're not listening to you. All they know is we are not giving them anything." I said, "They're desperate." He said, "Yes, they are, and if they are coming this way, we will have to take care of it." I looked straight ahead.

For 19 years, Cheryl worked at Memorial. When she earned her nursing degree from LSU in December 1987, she took a job the following month there (at the time, it was called Southern Baptist Hospital). She wanted to work in the SICU, but there were no vacancies. Newborn had an opening.

On Wednesday, August 31, Cheryl Barré is curled up on the windowsill in the education room of the women's unit. Another nurse wakes her. Moms and babies are leaving, now! Nurses are needed to accompany them, but they don't know how many. They will evacuate to Woman's Hospital in Baton Rouge, where the NICU babies have been brought. Cheryl tells her sister, a nurse who is also working at the hospital, that she may be leaving. Cheryl's sister has their father with her as well as her three children and husband.

At the women's unit, the nurses ready each mom. Each baby is placed in a sling and secured closely to its mother. Now the moms are hands-free and can use the hand rail for support. Cautiously, the nurses and the moms with babies make their way down six flights of stairs. Flashlights light the stairwell. A nurse positions herself behind each mother, while another nurse and dad are in front to prevent anyone from falling.

They reach the ER ramp, where several people wait to leave. The Plexiglas wall on the street side of the ramp has been knocked out. An airboat driver maneuvers his boat on the flooded street to the mid-section of the ER ramp. A physician in perspiration-soaked scrubs holds a rope tied to the boat. People step off the side of the ER ramp and board the airboat. Wads of cotton are in their ears to muffle the loud noise of the boat's fan engine.

"I am looking at those airboats and thinking, 'You have got to be kidding me. The babies will be deaf,' and they could not breathe with all of the wind from the engine," she says.

Cheryl hopes another boat comes soon. It will not be good to have these moms and babies retrace their steps upstairs. A flatboat pulls up with two young men. Growing up in south Louisiana, Cheryl has been in boats from a very young age. But she wonders how all the moms can fit in this one boat.

"We had open discussion on that ramp," says Cheryl. "All our NICU babies made it to Woman's Hospital. We are going to bring these moms and babies there. They are all no longer patients. Everyone is medically stable. We are going to find a family member or friend to get them in Baton Rouge. That was the plan."

Danielle, nurse manager of the nursery and lactation center, surveys the group of nurses from the women's unit. She turns to Cheryl.

"She said, 'Cheryl, you've got to go. You have MSK [medullary sponge kidney disease] and you have to stay hydrated all the time. You can't stay hydrated here.' Well, I know some nurses were upset and wanted to leave. I was fine to stay. Then someone yells they need an experienced nurse. One of the moms becomes extremely upset. I get in the boat and hand her baby to one of the men. I calm her down," recalls Cheryl.

The two men are volunteer firefighters from Houston. Cheryl sees that they are armed. Cheryl has heard of situations in the vicinity that were potentially violent. The moms feel reassured that the men are armed. One man is at the bow, the other at the stern. Cheryl sits in the middle, on the floor with the supplies. In front of her are two moms. Behind her are the other three.

The boat leaves the hospital. Cheryl looks back toward the hospital and sees her coworkers standing on the ER ramp. She is relieved the moms and babies are leaving. She feels regret leaving behind her fellow nurses.

The boat heads to South Claiborne Avenue and turns left toward Jefferson Parish. Downtown is 5 miles behind them. Once they reach their destination, Cheryl plans to hydrate and then return to the hospital to help with other evacuations.

"But for now I have to focus on the babies. The heat is sweltering," she says. "There is no shade, and the water splashes up from the motor. The water is so polluted. I asked them to slow it down a little bit. They probably thought I was crazy, asking to go slower to get out of there. I told the moms to keep those babies in the slings. We don't want to expose the babies to any of this splashing water. If it gets into their eyes or mouth it will be bad."

The boat continues its trek along Claiborne Avenue, passing Nashville Street, next Broadway. Then it hits ground. The men use poles to push the boat. It doesn't budge. They keep trying.

"Now we have all of this weight in that boat. I jumped out," she says. "The water touches the hem of my gym shorts. One guy yells, 'Ma'am, you don't have hip boots on!' They had waders on up to their chest. I tell him, 'Yes, I know, just come on.' I pulled the boat while they pushed from the back. Eventually it moved. They tell me to jump back in. I got back in, but banged the hell out of my left ankle getting in.

"People told me, 'You are going to see floating bodies. There is nothing you can do for these people,'" she continues. "Then we started

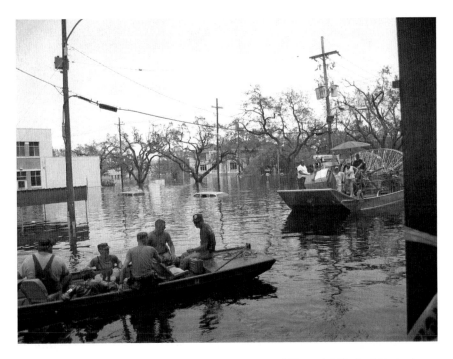

The National Guard leaves the emergency room ramp at Memorial Medical Center as a Wildlife and Fisheries boat arrives to evacuate patients. Photo by Sandra E. Cordray.

hearing people calling to us. 'Do you have any water?' People are in the trees on the avenue's neutral ground. They had come from their flooded homes. They are shouting, 'We need water, we need food.' I felt so bad, but we had nothing; only formula and diapers. One of the young guys said, 'Don't talk, ma'am. Look straight ahead. They're not listening to you. All they know is we are not giving them anything.' I said, 'They're desperate.' He said, 'Yes, they are, and if they are coming this way, we will have to take care of it.' I looked straight ahead. Some came out of the trees, but they were not getting any closer to us. They kept screaming louder. The mothers were crying at that point, and I told them, 'There is nothing to give them.' I kept looking straight ahead, and I'm thinking, 'If they try to tip this boat, these guys will be forced to do something and the moms are going to lose it.' I kept telling the mommas, 'Keep your babies covered, your mouth and eyes closed, because of the splashing water and just pray.' The babies are not making a sound. They are so overheated."

The boat reaches the railroad track, where several ambulances are lined up. Before leaving the boat, Cheryl takes out a fan. On the front is the company logo and a list of sister hospitals from a Mother's Day special event. The fans were given out to employees and volunteers to fan patients at the hot hospital. On her fan, she writes the names of the two men. Jack and D. J. They are brothers. Their father was part of the Wildlife and Fisheries group that helped evacuate flooded hospitals.

She thanks them. She sees a tent and recognizes another Memorial employee. A National Guard unit is there. Several elderly patients are sitting under the tent. Cheryl tells her colleague that they need to get the moms and babies to Baton Rouge. Cheryl hears that all the ambulances are going to Houston. Cheryl insists it has to be Baton Rouge. She is told there is no choice.

Cheryl directs her moms to the tent. The babies will have to get out of the heat. They are extremely lethargic. She directs the moms to stay under the tent and breast-feed their babies. "I tell them, 'If you are under the tent breast-feeding, no one is going to come around you.' One mom tells me she is bottle-feeding. I told her, 'Everything is contaminated. We can't even touch what we have brought with us. Just do it.' The elderly patients tell the Guardsmen, 'Let the mommas and the babies go. We can wait.' No telling how long they had been waiting."

For Cheryl, the only sign of organization is the straight line of ambulances. Everyone looks like a hospital patient. She walks toward the ambulances. As she walks down the row of ambulances, she glances at the number on the side of one vehicle. She knocks on a window. It rolls down.

Using their ambulance number, she inquires, "Are you ambulance number——? He says yes. I said, 'OK, you're for me. We have to take five mothers, five babies. Can you fit them?' He says, 'We can try.' I tell him, 'We are going to Woman's Hospital in Baton Rouge.' He says, 'No, we are going to Houston.' I say, 'Yes, but you have to go to Baton Rouge first. Then you are coming back to this line and going back home to Houston.' He said, 'All right.'

"I told him, 'I need you to pull out of that line and come closer and wait for us. I will bring the patients to you.' I told the moms to 'get up, follow me. Anyone talks to you, don't say a word. Just keep going.' I got all moms in the ambulance. I sat at the hull, at the head of the stretcher. It felt like the Arctic. I told them to turn the AC off. These babies are going to go into shock." Inside the ambulance, she checks each infant. Their core body temperatures are 100° plus. Once their body temperatures lower, they begin to suckle. She advises the driver that he can gradually turn on the AC. She tells the driver the babies are ready to go.

Cheryl is torn between accompanying the moms to Baton Rouge and returning to Memorial. There does not seem to be any room in the ambulance for her to squeeze in with them.

"The driver says, 'No way, get in here now,'" says Cheryl. "'We want a nurse who knows babies.' The moms are begging me to go with them. They know I want to get back to the hospital. I did not want to be the reason they didn't go to Baton Rouge."

Once inside the ambulance, she takes rubbing alcohol and wipes off the grime that covers her body. She tells the driver that in Baton Rouge, they will go LSU Tiger stadium, a familiar landmark. He does not know where that is. Unable to use the interstate, one mom knows a back way to Baton Rouge. They reach Woman's Hospital, where the staff is waiting outside for them. Cheryl thanks the ambulance drivers and tells them, "I hope you find your place back in that line. If not, just go back to Houston. You did your job."

On her fan she writes their names: Rick and Jeff.

The hospital staff usher Cheryl and the moms to a conference room, where there is food and water. Each of them has a hospital employee assigned to her, and they are each given a satellite phone so that they can call their families. Because she had been in the infested waters, Cheryl is taken to the showers for a decontamination scrubbing with alcohol foam.

She is given fresh scrubs. A nurse takes tennis shoes out of a locker. "She says, 'These are yours. That nurse is not on hurricane duty, so she won't need them,'" says Cheryl. "The staff at Woman's Hospital was incredible. They were a lifesaver to us."

In the conference room, she tries to find a friend or family member who can take each mom. One has family in Lafayette. They come and take her and another mom to their home. A third mom, in talking with a hospital employee, learns that they have a mutual friend. Another connection is made. Cheryl tells the last mom that if they can't find her family, Cheryl will stay with her. However, contact is made.

When the last mom leaves, Cheryl calls her hospital's headquarters to report the status of the moms and babies. The last person from Memorial left in the conference room, she tells the staff, "I need to go see the NICU babies from Memorial. Every baby had the card we had made and placed with them before they left our hospital. I said, 'It's very important that you leave that card on there, because when those mothers finally catch up with their babies, it will make them feel like 'I still know who my kid is.' Every baby is OK."

She sees a neonatologist from Memorial. He had accompanied one of the NICU babies on the helicopter flight to Woman's Hospital. He gives her a hug. She asks him whether, if she cannot find a way to contact her family, she can take a loan to get a taxi to Tunica, Mississippi, where her family evacuated. He tells her not to worry, he'll be around. Cheryl returns to the conference room. "I got teary-eyed. Do I go back to the hospital? They tell me this is a one-way ticket. You don't get to go back," she says.

Exhausted, Cheryl lies down in the ultrasound room. She talks with a technician who went to radiology school with her sister-in-law. Cheryl falls deeply asleep, until someone awakens her; standing there is her husband, Bryan. The hospital staff contacted him in Tunica. He has driven to Baton Rouge. He is recovering from recent surgery to implant a defibrillator. She learns that their home in St. Bernard Parish is gone. Bryan saw the peak of their roof, 3 feet above the floodwaters, on a satellite photo. The homes of everyone in her extended family are also gone. She is one of five children; her husband is one of six.

"But I didn't know that was going on. I was in a daze," explains Cheryl. "As we are leaving Woman's Hospital, a nurse gives me a lab coat. She tells me to check the pocket later. When I do, there is a $50 bill." Bryan takes Cheryl to Tunica, where she reunites with their three children and other family members. The next morning, they leave for Tennessee. The Barré family, 18 of them, stay in a condo for a few weeks. They need the time to make decisions. Cheryl discovers that her father and sister evacuated from Memorial via helicopter. They were dropped off on Interstate 10 and were put on a bus to Houston.

Cheryl finally speaks to her sister. On their way to Houston, Cheryl's sister contacted her husband's brother, who followed the bus. When the bus made a direction-finding stop, Joan and her immediate family got off. Her dad stayed on the bus, which took him to the Reliance Center, where relatives met him and brought him to Arlington, Texas, where his sisters and their children reside.

When Cheryl reaches her father, he tells her that their cousin has generously opened her home to them. Cheryl knows she needs to be close to her dad and leaves for Texas. She realizes she has to find a job. She calls her company's toll-free number. She finds a position at Trinity Medical Center in Carrollton, Texas.

"When we got to my cousin's house, I thought it was going to be awkward because I had not spoken to her in years," relays Cheryl. "But it was anything but awkward. Judy had welcome signs for us and gave us the upstairs."

After a few months of staying with her cousin, Bryan and Cheryl find a house nearby to rent. Weeks later, their family beagle, Princess, is found. Cheryl called a number from Petfinders.com, and it led to a veterinarian in Texas. The dog was discovered at Memorial by a Houston police officer, who was part of the search and rescue team. Princess was evacuated with other pets to NorthShore Regional Medical Center. The officer, who also had beagles, brought Princess on their missions. He put hospital bracelets on her paws and named her Katrina. He offered to adopt her if no one claimed her. Princess was placed in foster care with the vet in Aledo, Texas. His office was 20 minutes from Cheryl and Bryan's new home. Four months after Katrina, Princess comes home. The Barré children's other pet, a rat named Debra, was never found at the hospital.

Cheryl's commute to work is 1 hour 15 minutes. She works four night shifts a week. It is a major adjustment after 19 years of working the day shift, but she needs the job. Her second month at work, the hospital staff give her and a few other employees a post-Katrina shower. There are gifts of blankets, sheets, household items, and gift cards.

"That was just the nicest thing in the whole world. They totally absorbed me into their maternal–child family. This unit had a bulletin for personal photo displays. There were several categories of pictures.

I posted a photo of my house before and after Katrina. The post-Katrina picture shows my ceiling on the ground. Seaweed hangs from my ceiling fans. It was hard to tell which way was up on the picture. The picture said it all. The unit was great and the people were wonderful. I worked there until we returned to Louisiana." While in Texas, Cheryl quickly finds a medical network for her husband, who has a rare heart condition called arrhythmogenic right ventricular dysplasia (ARVD). After they get all the necessary medical tests for Bryan, they decide to be near family. They make plans to return to Louisiana in June 2006.

It is a seller's market, with so many displaced people relocating. Family members help Cheryl and Bryan search for a new house in Covington, 60 miles from their St. Bernard home. Bryan's sister sees a neighbor putting a for-sale sign in her yard. She asks the neighbor to hold off putting the sign out until she notifies Bryan and Cheryl. Through e-mailed photographs and phone conversations, they purchase the house. From their flooded home in St. Bernard, they retrieve a cement statue of the Virgin Mary, a Mother's Day present from several years before. They also find some pieces of china and a handful of muddy photos.

In June 2007, Cheryl begins working at a community hospital in St. Tammany Parish. Her home is less than 3 minutes from work. She says this hospital staff also greeted her with open arms and welcomed her into their maternal–child family. At work, she has met former patients from her nursing years at Memorial. One dad showed her a video of Cheryl admitting their first baby. He was thrilled that she was there for the birth of their second child.

Looking back at Hurricane Katrina and the hospital evacuation, Cheryl observes that nurses who are in nursing for what nursing really is can make a difference in any emergency, whether it is a hurricane, flood, earthquake, tornado, or any other catastrophe. People say it does not matter if you are there because they will always have emergency personnel to take care of things.

"I am here to tell you no! You and you alone can make a difference. When the time comes, you realize you are capable of doing things you never thought you would do." Cheryl hopes to find the ambulance drivers and volunteer firefighters who helped her bring the five moms and their babies to safety in Baton Rouge. "I wrote their names down on the fan so I wouldn't forget. I told my husband I need to track them down one day and tell them thank you. I will always remember what they did for us."

Danielle

People say it is actually worse than someone who goes to war because they expect something. I never expected when I went to work that all of this would happen and cause the end of my career. Because it is. It is the end of my patient care career.

Danielle RN, BSN, attended UNO and graduated from William Carey College School of Nursing in 1990. In 1989, while she was in her senior year of nursing school, she started her career at Baptist Hospital as a nurse tech for the women's division and remained there until 2005. During this time, she was employed as a staff nurse on the women's unit and in the newborn nursery. She later became an assistant manager in the newborn nursery and then manager of the newborn nursery and lactation center. Following Hurricane Katrina, she worked at a law firm reviewing medical records. She is currently employed at a New Orleans area hospital as a QA analyst and a corporate wellness nurse.

Ever since the fifth grade, Danielle wanted to be a nurse who took care of babies. So when she earned her nursing degree from William Carey College, she accepted a job at Southern Baptist Hospital (later named Memorial Medical Center) where she had worked as a nursing technician during her senior year of nursing school. For almost 17 years she was at the hospital for nearly every storm and flood, and even for the rare snowfall.

Now, on Sunday, August 28, Danielle, nurse manager of the newborn nursery and lactation center, arrived for work, bracing for another storm. In tow were her 22-month-old son and daughter who was approaching her fifth birthday. Her husband had planned to join the family but, delayed by boarding up their home in Metairie, he was forced to ride out the storm at their home.

On the sixth floor of Memorial Medical Center, Danielle surveys her unit to assess the well-baby newborns in the nursery. When the power goes out, the babies are stripped to their diapers to keep them cool in the hot summer air in the newborn nursery. By Tuesday morning, August 30, before the floodwaters arrive, one of the babies has left, when the family found an evacuation route not yet compromised by the rising floodwaters. Several of the parents stay in the nursery for hours at a time with the staff. It is as if they have become a part of the nursery staff family. "This made it difficult at times to keep the staff updated—not that I had much information to give them."

On Tuesday morning, patient evacuation plans are being discussed. Danielle says, "Two of the fathers became adamant about leaving. I told them there is news about a break in the levee, but no information on its location." One of the physicians receives word from his daughter, a medical reporter at one of the New Orleans television stations. She tells him the streets are like rivers.

Looking at the anxious men, Danielle understands why they want to take their families away to a safer place. She tells them she cannot prevent them from leaving but asks that they follow her to a room that has a view of Clara Street, bordering the hospital. She turns to them and says, " 'I want you to look at the street. And I want to tell you how quickly the water is rushing.' I think at that point it was up to a bumper. I said, 'I'd hate to think of you stranded on the street with a newborn baby and your wife who just had a C-section. She can't walk in the water.' "

One of the new dads is beside himself and breaks down. Danielle continues, "I am not telling you that you can't go. I am telling you to look at what you would be going into with a newborn, and who knows how far you can get."

The men acknowledge the gravity of the situation if they leave on their own. Back in the nursery, the mothers stay close to the staff. Danielle knows they want more information, but she has no answers for them. She says, "I helped with the preparation for evacuating the babies in the NICU." Late Tuesday, when the NICU babies are safely evacuated via helicopter to Woman's Hospital in Baton Rouge, the staff is elated.

On Wednesday morning, Danielle goes downstairs to the ER entrance and speaks to the manager of the operating room, who indicates that all the babies have been successfully evacuated. Danielle shouts back, "No, they're not!"

Danielle immediately goes back to the newborn nursery to help the staff prepare the babies for evacuation. She provides instructions to the staff and states, "Only one bag will be allowed, which will contain essential supplies for the babies." A nurse goes to the lactation center to obtain slings, which will help with the evacuation of the babies. "We use the slings to help carry the babies. We will take the babies and their mothers to the stairs to the ER." The babies are gently placed in the slings that hold them snugly to their moms. This way, the mothers have their arms free, yet their babies are close and secure. Formula and diapers for each newborn are packed to fit in each mom's personal bag.

Waiting on the ER ramp, Danielle and her nurses decide that if only one nurse can leave, it will be their colleague Cheryl. She has a medical condition now compromised by the heat that soars above 110° inside the hospital.

"We were concerned with the dehydration. Those of us on the ER ramp agreed if only one person, she would go. And that is what ended up . . . what happened. They only wanted one nurse to go. She went with the five mothers. And she went a different path," explains Danielle.

"The mothers and babies are seated in chairs on the ER ramp, waiting for their boat (it could not be an airboat—the noise could rupture their eardrums)." Then one of the mothers says, "Let's take a picture." The nurse obliges. The mom is trying to cheer the others and takes photos so that there will be a reminder of when they left. "You were doing it because it was making some of them feel better," says Danielle, whose focus is on the pending evacuation for babies and moms.

Danielle says, "After the boat leaves, all of us on the ER ramp begin to cry and hug each other. We are so relieved that the babies are gone, but scared of what would happen. When would we get to go?"

Realizing that the fathers will have to leave in a separate boat becomes a concern for Danielle "because the emotions of those mothers leaving their husbands were phenomenal. The next big quest was to round up all my dads and get them on a boat."

To do so, Danielle knows they cannot be seen as "cutting to the front of the line," as 4 days at the hospital have frayed nerves. Danielle positions the five dads and a grandmother among the employees and volunteers who are fanning the patients waiting on the ER ramp. The ramp has become a docking area for boats that are ferrying people away from the hospital.

The grandmother, who cannot speak much English, is sobbing. Her son-in-law, concerned that the elderly woman will be left behind because the fathers are leaving, tells Danielle he cannot leave the woman. Danielle quietly assures him that they both will leave. She puts her fingers to her lips and motions the woman to be quiet. A boat approaches the side of the ER ramp. It slams hard against the side, where Plexiglas hangs. There is a crash, and a sheet of glass comes down. Miraculously, no one is injured.

The dads and the elderly woman board a boat and leave. Danielle is relieved they are gone and tells herself, "Now I have to just get the other people I feel responsible for out."

On Wednesday, August 31, around 6:00 P.M., Danielle leaves Memorial Medical Center. Her son's condition has not improved. She steps onto a waiting boat, holding him. He is lethargic; he has developed impetigo. "I was very torn about leaving when all of my staff had not yet been evacuated, but I had to get him to a better place," Danielle recounts. Two of her nurses (one to help her with her children and another who had become ill) leave with her. The director of hospital plant operations, is steering his boat, which he brought to the hospital. At the bow is the director of hospital security. Danielle asks them what is their destination. They reply that they have directions to bring evacuees as close as they can to St. Charles and Napoleon avenues. From there, buses will take them to a shelter on the West Bank or in Baton Rouge. Danielle's hopes soar. Danielle has friends and relatives in Baton Rouge.

The boat stops. The water is too shallow to continue. Danielle and the others on the boat step off into the flooded street and walk toward St. Charles Avenue in the knee-deep water. People mill about. There seems to be no organization, no one from the hospital. There are no resources. She turns back to where the boat was. It is gone. It has returned to the hospital.

She overhears a nurse talking about going to the Elms Mansion on St. Charles Avenue, about a mile away. Danielle stands nearby. Perhaps they can hitch a ride with her. She tries to call her family. After a few unsuccessful tries, she reaches her in-laws in Atlanta. Her father-in-law tells her that her husband evacuated earlier in the day and is safe in Baton Rouge. Danielle's dad and father-in-law had convinced her husband that it was not safe to stay and thought she would be safe at the hospital. Danielle asks her father-in-law if he can find out if one of their friends has stayed at a home nearby so she can contact him; the friend had also evacuated to Baton Rouge.

By now, two nurses and their families have joined Danielle. A school bus passes, crammed with passengers. An 18-wheeler flatbed truck stops near the intersection. People climb aboard. No one can tell them where the truck is going. They just want to leave and find shelter. One of the husbands tells Danielle's group that they all need to board one of the vehicles. Night is coming. It will not be safe to stay on the street.

The Audubon Zoo mobile pulls up. They board. There is standing room only. Someone asks, "Where are we going?"

Danielle says, "You just got on the bus and you couldn't tell where you were going because it's dark and you're standing. You're not at the front of the bus where you can see where you are going. So you had no idea. Then all of a sudden, it is like, oh, my God! We are at the Convention Center!"

The following is from Robert Siegel's National Public Radio "All Things Considered" interview with Michael Chertoff, Secretary of Homeland Security, and John Burnett reporting from Ernest N. Morial Convention Center, September 1, 2005 (Kennedy, 2005).

SIEGEL: We are hearing from our reporter—and he's on another line right now—thousands of people at the Convention Center in New Orleans with no food, zero.

CHERTOFF: As I say, I'm telling you that we are getting food and water to areas where people are staging. And, you know, the one thing about an episode like this is if you talk to someone and you get a rumor or you get someone's anecdotal version of something, I think it's dangerous to extrapolate it all over the place. The limitation here on getting food and water to people is the condition on the ground. And as soon as we can physically move through the ground with these assets, we're going to do that. So—

SIEGEL: But Mr. Secretary, when you say that there is—we shouldn't listen to rumors, these are things coming from reporters who have not only covered many, many other hurricanes; they've covered wars and refugee camps. These aren't rumors. They're seeing thousands of people there.

CHERTOFF: Well, I would be—actually I have not heard a report of thousands of people in the Convention Center who don't have food and water. I can tell you that I know specifically the Superdome, which was the designated staging area for a large number of evacuees, does have food and water. I know we have teams putting food and water out at other designated evacuation areas. So, you know, this isn't—and we've got plenty of food and water if we can get it out to people. And that is the effort we're undertaking.

BURNETT: Let me clarify for the secretary and for everyone else . . . just drove away from three blocks from here in the Ernest Morial Convention Center. There are, I estimate 2,000 people living like animals inside the city convention center and around it. They've been there since the hurricane. There's no food. There's absolutely no water. There's no medical treatment. There's no police and no security. And there are two dead bodies lying on the ground and in a wheelchair beside the Convention Center, both elderly people, both covered with blankets now. We understand that two other elderly people died in the last couple of days. We understand that there was a 10-year-old girl who was raped in the Convention Center in the last two nights. People are absolutely desperate there. I've never seen anything like this.

The Convention Center spans several city blocks along Convention Center Boulevard, which runs parallel to the Mississippi River. It is nine city blocks from the Superdome, where thousands of people have taken shelter from the hurricane. Danielle steps off the bus. There are no police, no military personnel. No one seems to be in charge. People mill about in pockets of groups. Danielle recognizes, from a distance, a nurse from the nursery and a technician from the hospital. Her husband tells them there is a cooler place inside the Convention Center. He and another spouse go inside to check it out. They return and report that it appears safe for the night.

They enter the cavernous Convention Center and are stunned by what they see. This is not a shelter. It is a place of anarchy.

"People had taken over the scooters and golf carts; they're racing with them. If you didn't get out of their way they would roll over you. The only lights were from people who had flashlights. I remember there was someone not too far from us who had candles on an ice chest, and I am thinking, 'We are going to die in a fire.' They were selling drugs. They had broken into the concession stands and they were trying to sell you the alcohol," she says.

Danielle and the others settle next to a column in one of the sections of the Convention Center. They sit down, forming a serpentine shape around the column. They count their supplies. In her one bag, Danielle has diapers and important papers. She also has two bottles of water and two small packs of peanut butter crackers. They talk about how they are going to get out. One of them reaches a family member on her cell phone. They have a relative in the military who is prepared to drive to the city with his comrades and rescue them. A nurse's husband works for Outback Restaurant. Danielle's father-in-law, in Atlanta, reaches the husband's supervisor, whose boss is willing to bring in meals to the Convention Center. The plan is that they will get into the back of the van while the meals are distributed. Another call is made. Danielle's brother's National Guard Reserve unit will do an unauthorized rescue mission.

Exhausted they try to sleep, but in shifts so that a few stand watch. Danielle tries to get her son to sleep. He begins crying. Another child cries. A stranger approaches their group and threatens that if they can't stop the crying they will come back and shut up the children. Danielle shoves her son against her armpit to muffle his cries. On Wednesday night, someone was calling out for help for an older woman. They had no supplies, and they could do nothing.

During the night somebody dies near them. A group of adults and teens put the body on a cart that is used to move tables and chairs. They parade the body around the Convention Center Hall. The Convention Center seems to be in the hands of hoodlums who patrol the area. They shout obscenities and randomly select who they will threaten next. Sounds of gun shots ring out and people scramble away from the windows toward Danielle and her friends. She fears they will be trampled. The "gun fire" turns out to be only firecrackers. It is nearing 3:00 A.M. Someone shouts that buses have arrived. Seven Coach chartered buses pull up by the sidewalk in front of the center. Danielle says her group does not leave. It is best to let the mob leave first. But no one leaves "because people acted like animals," she explains. "They jumped on the bus and were rocking them back and forth. The drivers can't blame them, drove off." On Thursday morning, September 1, the group moves to another section in the Convention Center. It seems to be no better than where they were before. A man comes up to the group. He asks for help finding his wife. She worked in the radiology department at Memorial Medical Center. If they help him find her, he will help them find a way out. Danielle and a few others canvas the area for the man's wife. "When I got back from doing that search, they tell me, 'OK, Danielle, some people have figured out some of us were in scrubs. There was a lady who was pregnant who was having contractions. We told her you need to be on your left side. Keep hydrated. There wasn't anything else we could do.'"

A National Guard unit drives by the Convention Center. The soldiers have their guns pointed toward the crowd. The soldiers do not stop. Danielle and the others talk softly about how they can escape. They cannot survive on their meager rations. Danielle rations the water and food for her children. "You tell them to take a sip of water and you could see your child wants more. You had to pull the bottle back and watch their little lips shake. I didn't eat. I let my kids eat. I did eat one peanut butter cracker. It was on the floor. I wasn't going to eat it, but I said, 'Oh well, I'll eat it.' One girl had a bag of Tootsie Roll pops, which she gave to everybody. She said, 'Let's keep our blood sugar up.' Two guys said, 'Well, people already broke into the concession,' so they went and got a container of soft drink syrup for the sugar. Iced tea syrup doesn't taste good. Sprite's a little bit better."

Cell phones stop working inside the Convention Center. They go outside and try to make calls. Sitting on the street curb, they see a New Orleans police car drive along Convention Center Boulevard. Two of the nurses approach the car. They wave their hospital badges to get the officers' attention. They want to see if the police can increase their drive-by visits. Maybe it will calm the crowd inside. One officer looks at the nurses and says, "Lady, get on the curb, or I am going to shoot you."

By now, Danielle says, their group has been noticed by others. Outside, they try to call again. There are more threats.

"You think you're better than us, you're going to get out of here before us. We're the law. We are going to take care of you tonight," relates Danielle.

Danielle's mother-in-law had called the hospital's parent company to tell them that several of their employees are stranded at the Convention Center. She works in the travel industry and has been trying to reach nearby hotels. If Danielle and the others can walk to a hotel, will they give them shelter? There is no reply from the hotels. Danielle reaches the corporate office for Memorial Medical Center. A representative tells her that buses are on their way. Some of Danielle's colleagues share this news with the people threatening them, "buses are coming, but you have to tell your people if they behave like they behaved last night the buses are not going to stay."

Danielle begins, "People had urinated and defecated all over the place. Not even in the bathroom, just wherever. You'd see people being sexually assaulted right in front of you."

Another sliver of hope comes to them. A Memorial Medical Center nurse, receives a text from her husband. He has contact with the St. Charles Parish Sheriff's Office. If she and the others can walk across the Crescent City Connection and reach the toll booths, the officers will be there. Otherwise, the St. Charles Parish Sheriff's Office would have to cross three jurisdictional boundaries to reach them at the Convention Center. The group discusses this option at length. They see what they can discard from their bags to lighten their load. A shopping cart can be used to move the children. There is another cart they can use. If anyone needs to stop and rest, all of them will stop. They start walking. But after a few yards, many of them are out of breath. Weak, they cannot go any farther. Then they see people walking down the bridge ramp by the Convention Center. Danielle feels her heart race. The situation has become surreal. She looks at her colleagues.

"Here I am," she recalls. "I have postpartum and nursery nurses and their families, and I am a manager. 'I am one of the people who made you come [to work]. . . . I think I am going to have a heart attack.' They said, 'No, you are having a panic attack. Get yourself to relax.' Later, when we were out of there, one of my nurses, she told me, 'I thought we were fine because you were fine. When you had that panic attack,' she said, 'I thought, this is not good. Thank God you came out of it.'"

The group from Memorial are still hopeful that buses will come. A man in a blue uniform begins directing the crowd. No one knows who he is with, but people seem to listen to him. Single lines form as the crowd waits for the buses. Danielle notices that she and her group are being watched by the people they had told earlier to behave because buses were coming. As they sit and wait, they are joined by another nurse from Memorial and her sister. Two Australian girls from Brisbane, carrying luggage, befriend them as well. Their flight arrived in New Orleans on Saturday, August 27. They were staying at the Monteleone Hotel on Poydras Street. The hotel arranged for buses to evacuate hotel guests, but city officials commandeered them to use at the Superdome. The tourists had tried to walk across the Crescent City Connection to the other side of the river but were turned back.

There are now 28 in Danielle's group. Hours pass, and they wait for the buses. "There was one gentleman who came up to us. He said that he didn't agree with all the looting that was going on. He had a couple of breakfast bars that he gave to the kids, which was very nice. And then after a while it became very apparent that no buses were coming. People in our area that we had told that buses were coming were very angry toward us. Two women tried to give us a large bottle of Kentwood water. There was almost a riot. . . . These two women were saying, 'Let them have the water.' Finally, we said, 'We don't want the water.' At that point, we decided that it would not be safe to go back into the Convention Center for the night. That if they did indeed follow through with their threats, we'd be trapped. We crossed the street. They sent people, who positioned themselves close to us so that they could hear what we were saying."

One of the Memorial nurse's cell phone has one bar left. She sends her husband one final text message.

"She was saying her good-byes," Danielle pauses. Her voice waivers. "At that point she gets a text from her sister. She is told to go underneath the overpass and to wait for somebody from the sheriff's department to find her, but she needs to be alone. Two men in our group follow to ensure her safety. They were gone for quite some time."

One of the Memorial nurses reaches the site. A man walks up to her and tells her, "Lady, it's not good for you to be here." She replies that she is trying to find somebody. He inquires if she has people with her and if they have food. The reply is, "Yes, some food." Then the stranger gives her a box of cereal—Cinnamon Toast Crunch—and walks away.

At the Convention Center, hours pass. The group believes that their colleague made her connection and will not be returning. The next day is Friday. Danielle lies back with her son on her chest; he is extremely lethargic. His skin is clammy and cold. Danielle shrugs her shoulders several times to startle him. He does not respond. She asks another Memorial nurse to check his pulse another nurse, to check his pulse and respiration because she cannot feel his breath. The nurse finds his pulse. It is very low.

They begin talking out loud so the thugs will hear them. "We start saying how we were staying over on this side because it was cooler, there was some starlight, it was good for the kids, that we were going to be sleeping in shifts to let them know we're not going to sleep," Danielle says.

The group camps out across from the Convention Center. From the darkness, a car drives by. The window is rolled down. There is a voice. "Are y'all OK? Do you need any help?" Danielle says that at first, they were immobilized hearing that someone wanted to know if they were OK.

"Finally, one of the Memorial nurses got up and went over to the car and told him who we were. He says, 'We are looking for you. We are St. Charles Parish Sheriff's Department. Go lie down, do not make a big to-do, but you need to be ready to go, we will be back around midnight.' And shortly after they drove away, René came back. She is beside herself, hysterical, crying, 'They never came! They never came!' We tried to inconspicuously tell her, 'They did, they did come.' So we lie down, ready to go. I had both kids, so I asked René, 'I need you to help me with my daughter to get to the bus because they said you will have to run to the bus.' All of a sudden it was like they were there because they came in without their headlights and you didn't know there was a black car. You didn't even know there was a car in front of you, then all of a sudden there is a flashlight, and we hear like, 'Get up and go!' So we are running to the corner. We ran to the end of Convention Center Boulevard, which was several blocks, and then you took that right close to the bridge on-ramp. We are running and I remember getting to the curb on the corner and

I could hear their radios go off. . . . 'Tell them to run! Tell them to run! We can't hold them off anymore! Make them run!'"

"I remember getting to the bus and trying to get up the steps . . . being so weak, trying to hurry so everybody could get on the bus, falling up the steps then sitting in the backseat of the bus. I looked at my fellow nurse and said, 'Where is my daughter?' And she said she was dead weight. She couldn't carry her. 'I gave her to a policeman. I think I gave her to a policeman!'"

Terror grips Danielle. She hands her son to someone and shouts that she needs to get off the bus. An officer tries to calm her and asks her to describe the child. The bus is now filling with others that were in the group. As they hear that Danielle's daughter is missing, their anguish is palpable to everyone. Another officer does a head count. Then Danielle hears someone on a radio. "Yes, we have a curly-haired blonde. She is in the back of the SUV."

The bus and police cars drive away from the Convention Center. At the top of the bridge on-ramp, they stop. There is another head count. An officer asks who was inquiring about the curly-headed blonde. They raise her up so that Danielle can see her daughter. "Later, she asked me, 'How come they raised me up?' 'Because you weren't sitting by me and I needed to see you,'" recalls Danielle. The officers, clad in bulletproof vests, are fully armed. Danielle says they had brought enough ammunition to take on a small country. When they thought a child had been left behind, they were planning how to go back and get her.

The convoy drives west. They bring everyone to St. Charles Parish Hospital for triage. In the ER, intravenous fluids are ordered for her son. Danielle begs them not to start the intravenous infusion and see if he will drink. He does.

"We got into the cafeteria after everybody else had been there. They fed you. We talked about it later, all of us that were there, how we were hoarding food because they had a big feast and we were stuffing food in our pockets like it wasn't over yet. For weeks my daughter would say she didn't need a bottle of water, that we can all drink out of one. My son would just walk up to anybody and start eating off their plate."

Danielle is given a satellite phone to call her family. She reaches her mother-in-law. The only words that she is able to say are, "We got out." The St. Charles Parish sheriff's wife tells Danielle's mother-in-law where they are.

It has taken time for Danielle and her children to process the experience. "For a brief point in time, we were completely numb. Surely all of this didn't happen to me. It has taken a while. It hasn't all gone away. The other day, I had to bring my son on a field trip across the lake, and I have to drive across the lake to one of the clinics I work at once a month. Driving on the Causeway did not bother me before, but now I always get on the phone; I don't like getting on that bridge because you are surrounded by water.

"As I am bringing him on the field trip, I was thinking, 'He is in the back.' Surely talking to him is enough, and I was like, 'Oh, my God.' It overtook me and I had to pull over in one of those crossovers. We are sitting there, and he asked, 'What's wrong.' 'Oh, I am having a moment! Not feeling good. Just have to wait a second.' It's like, I've got my phone ready, who do I call, who do I know would answer the phone? Who could talk to me?

"I don't think you realize what situation you'll be in. People say it is actually worse than someone who goes to war because they expect something. I never expected when I went to work that all of this would have happened and cause the end of my career. Because it is. It is the end of my patient care career. At this point in time, I am not willing to work in a storm. I trust no one. When people say it won't happen again, well, I never would have thought it would have happened to begin with. Your longevity. You had so much trust in the place that you were, to be someplace new? No. And then to see my children. My daughter will ask me, do I miss the babies? Yes, I do. Except if I were with the babies, if there was a storm, I would have to work and you would go. And she breaks into tears. And I tell her, 'That's why I do what I do now.'"

Her son has no memory of the ordeal, but her daughter remembers. She does not talk about it as much anymore.

Her mother recounts, "When we were waiting for the buses that never came, a woman was yelling at some boys, telling them she wanted them to behave. Her daughter asked me if the National Guardsmen or the police shot her because she acted up. I told her, 'I think she was trying to stress to them that they needed to behave.'"

In 2007, there was an emotional reunion with the St. Charles Parish Sheriff's Office. It was the home of the department's public information officer, who wrote about their rescue in his book *Chest Deep and Rising: The Hurricane Katrina Nightmare*. Danielle brings a trophy. "We had a plaque made with all of their names on it for their heroic rescue," she says.

"I think the ties with everybody we used to work with, we still keep in touch, but the people that you went through that portion with, you can't let those go."

Four years later, Danielle tries to comprehend the behaviors she witnessed at the Convention Center.

"What I can't understand is why people had to behave the way they did. They stole barbeque pits and were grilling the food that they stole from Walmart. You had people coming in saying how it was going to be a better Christmas this year with TVs and what they were stealing. Where do you think you're taking it? They won't let you on the bus with that! What is going through your mind as opposed to how are we going to get out of here? How to maintain the people you're with, that was not the mentality of the people around us. There were some people that were nice, and I remember somebody offered us some cold cuts and we were so afraid. We didn't know if it was safe, so we said no, thank you, we're good. There were some genuine people there, but those people were so overshadowed by the people that could not control themselves."

Danielle has tried to share her experience with others in the hope that she could broaden their understanding of what to expect in the aftermath of a catastrophe. However, she feels that many have a false confidence that they are prepared for a catastrophic event.

"They think they're OK, and they don't need to hear what you might want to share with them. I was like, 'You need to get flashlights that you can wear on your head,' and they're like, 'We're good.' . . . And I'm thinking, 'But that's not how you should think anymore.' They think their facility did fine in Katrina . . . they were not surrounded by water. Who would have thought this is what would have happened?"

5 Pendleton Memorial Methodist Hospital

As early as 1960, there had been discussions between Kenneth Schor and Reverend John Koelemay about the dire need for a hospital to serve the eastern New Orleans area (Methodist Health System Foundation Inc. [MHSF], 2008). Seven years later, Pendleton Lahde opened Pendleton Memorial Methodist Hospital on property donated by George Williams, a community leader of Metairie, and the late Bill James of Ruston, Louisiana. Mr. Pendleton was the original board member and benefactor of the hospital and was instrumental in paving the way for many donors. The site selected was located on the eastern side of the Industrial Canal so that the underserved area of Gentilly and East Gentilly could receive medical care. Construction began on the hospital in 1967, and the first patient was admitted in 1968. The hospital was a 181-bed facility that added several services over the years, including a Psychiatric Pavilion, Advanced Surgery Center, and Home Health Services.

The hospital was used by patients from eastern New Orleans for over 35 years, when there was no Interstate 10 and when people died because the closest hospital was many miles away, or the Industrial Canal bridge was in the "up" position (MHSF, 2008). Following the current trend for large proprietary chains to acquire or merge with not-for-profit hospitals, majority ownership of Pendleton Memorial Methodist Hospital was sold to Universal Health Services (UHS) in 2003. As a result of the sale of the hospital to UHS, the Legacy Foundation (the Methodist Health System Foundation Inc.), a faith-based health care system, was established and retained 10% ownership. The foundation continues to serve people in the greater New Orleans area, with an emphasis on St. Bernard, New Orleans East, and Gentilly, to improve health care and health disparities (MHSF, 2008).

Methodist was severely damaged by Hurricane Katrina and has not been open since the last person was evacuated from the hospital on September 3, 2005. In 2006, New Orleans secured legislation that would allow for the operation of Methodist as a community hospital.

On May 26, 2009, Champion Medical Center (an independent medical center) opened in New Orleans East; it was founded and funded by Gregory Davis, who used $250,000 to build a 1,600-square-foot primary health care clinic from scratch at 9890 Lake Forest Boulevard. Davis was a professional boxer who was inspired to open the clinic when he had to drive several miles to bring his daughter to the closest open hospital.

In September 2009, the Orleans Parish Hospital Service District continues to work toward the purchase of the closed Methodist Hospital and to secure financing to put it back in service.

The incredible stories of three nurses who placed their lives on the line as they cared for the patients, families, and coworkers at Methodist Hospital before, during, and after the storm highlight the attributes and character of these outstanding nurses.

Michelle Pearson

I knew if I went to bed someone would die and I couldn't do that. Adrenalin is a great drug. That's what kept me alive, my adrenalin.

Michelle Pearson, RN, BSN, graduated from Louisiana State University Health Sciences Center in 2003 with a bachelor of science in nursing. She accepted a position at Methodist Hospital in New Orleans East as a critical care registered nurse. After Katrina, in 2005, she moved with her husband to Jackson, Tennessee, and became the director of a progressive care unit for 1 year, then an intensive care unit (ICU) director for 2 years. Currently she is working as an RN in a medical, surgical, and cardiac ICU.

Michelle was familiar with hospital evacuation for storms. In late September 2004, Hurricane Ivan had reached Category 5 strength. At its peak, Ivan was the size of the state of Texas and threatened southeast Louisiana, prompting evacuation. More than one-third of the greater New Orleans population left the city. On September 16, Hurricane Ivan made landfall in Gulf Shores, Alabama, as a Category 3 storm. It caused an estimated $133 billion in damages to the United States.

Prior to that landfall, Methodist Hospital coordinated its patient evacuation through the hospital's parent company, UHS. Patients were taken to a sister hospital in Lake Charles, Louisiana, due west of New Orleans. Michelle recalls a smooth evacuation and was notified of the plans before she reported to work. Nursing units packed supplies needed to take care of the patients. Half the patients traveled by ground ambulance, the rest by air. Families drove to Lake Charles. Three days later, military transport helicopters were used for the return to New Orleans. Michelle accompanied her patients by ambulance.

One year later, in 2005, Michelle expects a similar scenario to unfold at the hospital as it prepares for Hurricane Katrina. The 194-bed hospital has a 36-bed ICU that provides care for medical, cardiac, and surgical intensive care patients.

The Friday night before the storm, Michelle goes through her home in Chalmette and packs a 3-day supply of clothes and food. She also relocates wedding shower gifts to high shelves in closets. Plans are set for an October wedding, and half her invitations have been mailed. Her mother and fraternal twin sister have evacuated to Lafayette, Louisiana, a 3-hour drive southwest of New Orleans. As her fiancé packs additional belongings to take to his mother's home in Tennessee, he cannot hide his concerns from Michelle. "He was a nervous wreck," recalls Michelle. "He told me he thought that he was leaving me behind to die. I told him, 'It's my job. I have got to go. If nobody else is going to show up, who is going to take care of the patients?' And he understood that. That is my job. My duty. And when I became a nurse, I have to work holidays, I have to work disasters. He knows."

Now, alone in her house, Michelle listens to the latest update on the storm. New Orleans is in the center of its path. She calls the hospital. She is to report Sunday morning for work. She inquires, "Are there plans to evacuate the hospital?" There is no word about evacuation. She calls again on Saturday. She asks, "What are the evacuation plans?" The reply is that there will be no evacuation. Michelle is stunned. She watches the storm tracking on the news. A sinking feeling comes over her.

"At that point, I knew we are going to be underwater," she states. "I knew it was going to happen. I thought they didn't want to spend the money. They spent a lot of money the last time they evacuated. I felt, 'OK, we are going to be in trouble.' I didn't think we were going to be in that much trouble! I knew we were going to lose electricity. I didn't think the water was going to go up like that. It was scary. I knew I had to go into work and take care of these patients."

As she heads for work on Sunday at 6:30 A.M., she is the only one on her street who stayed. There are no cars on the road as she drives to the hospital. "I was very scared. My mom kept calling me and checking on me. You roam your house and think, 'What can I put up high enough? What do I want to have when I come back?' I tried to rearrange stuff. I put my vases in the bathroom, thinking that would cushion them. I had a rough night. I was upset, so as soon as I arrived at the hospital, I started crying. I had just bought a car, knowing that my car was going to be swept away with water."

Her colleagues also believed there would be an evacuation. It is hard for them to hide their anxiety. That evening, they are informed that the hospital is standing in place because of the mayor's request for area hospitals to remain open. "I don't know the main reason and I probably never will. I don't think any of us ever will," says Michelle. By the end of the day, Methodist Hospital is full of patients, employees, and family of both groups. People from the community drop off their family members—a mother, or grandmothers. Says Michelle, "They dropped them off for us to take care of and then left. We had a lot of those, some from a nursing home and the vent-dependent patients. We couldn't turn them away."

"We had a good amount of doctors. We had some great doctors over there. They were unbelievable, what these people did, in my eyes."

On Monday, by 7:00 A.M., the storm bears down on Methodist Hospital. Anticipating loss of water, employees fill garbage cans and any other open containers. The ICU on the second floor has a circular floor plan with an elevator in the middle. A nursing station is on each side. The area is surrounded by windows. Michelle describes the unit as "gorgeous, but perhaps not practical for hurricane-force winds." As the winds bear down on the hospital, the windows burst in the ICU. There is a staccato popping sound as the glass breaks. Quickly, the staff move the patients in their beds from the unit to the protected doorway. Nurses use their bodies and pillows as shields to protect their patients from the flying glass.

"We pulled them out of the room to the doorway as far as the oxygen line to the wall would reach, and we covered them. The nurses—we weren't thinking about ourselves. We wanted to take care of the patients. I remember covering my patient with my whole body. Each nurse had four patients to watch."

And as quickly as the storm arrives, the winds leave. Michelle hears the generators start. The patients are wheeled back into the ICU. A maintenance crew arrives to board up the areas that are now gaping holes. Some are left alone to bring in more ventilation—a reprieve from the August heat. Ice packs help the patients cope with the soaring temperatures. Michelle says it is sunny outside. From their second-floor unit, she and her colleagues then notice the rising water. On the top is a film of fuel and household waste. The nearby Murphy Oil Refinery is among the storm's casualties. Michelle describes the water as "disgusting. It just kept coming up. I kept watching the letters on a sign at this window for the cancer center across the street—that was my waterline. It kept going higher and higher. Then finally, Tuesday afternoon, it had stopped rising."

The water is chest high. The hospital parking lot is a lake with submerged cars. Residents who had not evacuated crawl slowly to the pitch of their houses' roofs. The hospital's first floor, where pharmacy, lab, and radiology are located, is flooded. The water inches halfway up the walls. More patients come to the ICU—these are from the Health Care South Rehabilitation Unit, whose roof collapsed.

Hospital resources are nearing maximum capacity, as more people find their way to the hospital by boat or by swimming. Some enter by a stairwell next to the ICU. Some walk unannounced through the ICU. The staff tend to their cuts. By Wednesday, August 31, a more formal triage system is in place. Some people have superficial scratches from tree branches and wounds to their heads or arms. In the distance, a Coast Guard helicopter drops a basket to rescue someone from a rooftop.

Communications are vague about a rescue timeline. "They said, 'Oh, yes, they'll be here.' I thought they would be here Monday night, but nothing," says Michelle. "You look out the window and you are surrounded by water. You see a couple of boats, maybe the Coast Guard with a basket, but that's about it. There was nothing. It was just dead. You're in the slumps now."

There are no shift changes. Nurses work almost nonstop. Michelle does not sleep that Sunday through Thursday. She does not eat, but she sips water to keep hydrated. "I knew if I went to bed someone would die, and I couldn't do that," she explains. "Adrenalin is a great drug. That's what kept me alive, my adrenalin," she adds.

"I brought a big duffle bag of food and water. . . . We had so many people in the hospital that they were trying to gather up food to hand out. I gave them my bag. They had food in our break room, but the doors and windows were all open. I could see the family members in the lobby. We had a lot of children in the hospital, too, and they were sitting out in the waiting room. I felt so bad—'Here, have it all. Take my food, take my water—I will get some eventually.' I really wasn't thinking about food and water. At the time, you are thinking, 'How is this person's blood pressure, how am I going to run upstairs to where they moved pharmacy, get the medicine, and come back, and hopefully his blood pressure didn't drop.'

"It's over 100°, and you didn't want food and water. You wanted to take care of the patients and get out." Generator power is becoming a concern. To ration diesel fuel, the plan is to turn off the generators for periods of time throughout the day. It is imperative that the nurses remain at the bedside to hand-bag the patients. They do so for 8 or 12 hours, rotating turns with administrators, physicians, some members of the New Orleans Police Department, and a few military personnel who are embedded at the hospital.

Michelle sees snakes and an alligator in the waters. A nutria is trapped in the stairwell, unable to find a way out. A few people, finding the confinement of the hospital to be too much, leave. One jumps into the water. "I am sure something happened to them," says Michelle. "You had those incidents where people just lost it; would do anything to just get out of the hospital, including jumping into the water where the alligators were. "You see all of that, then you hear the gunshots, and you have (to worry about) people trying to get to the Pyxis machine for the narcotics."

One of the dialysis nurses creates "Katrinawear" as a diversion from the direness of their situation. She cuts off the sleeves and the legs of the nurses' scrubs because of the sweltering heat. "She would give nurses hand massages and offer to wash their hair. She just made light of it and she said, 'You know what? Why do we have to suffer?'" says Michelle.

The husband of the ICU medical director uses his boat to find more supplies. The hospital maintenance staff take a boat to find more bottled water. On their return, they unload their goods in buckets, which are lifted to a window near the ICU. The supplies are organized on a table and allocated for each floor.

"Wednesday the sewer started backing up. You had all those factors, and then you had patients, and there is no ice, no air-conditioning. They all had fevers, temperatures are rising. There is nothing you can do.

What can you do?" says Michelle. "You can give Tylenol so many times, but if their gut's not working, it's not going to absorb the Tylenol. . . . I felt very, very frustrated. I thought we would have been out of there by then. I really did. I kept saying, 'Oh, today's the day we all get out of here.' But you know what? We still have tons of people in the hospital, nobody has been evacuated. By that point, our flashlights are running out. At nighttime, it's pitch dark. You can't see anything. You can't document because you can't see. The stairwell, when you are trying to get to pharmacy, is pitch black. You don't know what's behind each corner. It's a scary situation."

Media reports fuel the frustration. "I didn't have time to sit down and listen," says Michelle. "The reports I was getting focused on Charity Hospital and the gunshots and stuff like that. I was telling myself, 'Just get us out of here.' We were running out of supplies, we had no water. Let's get out of here. We can't bag 24/7 trying to keep these patients alive. We are running out of energy. I did hear one report that said Methodist Hospital was totally evacuated. Oh, imagine that, we are still here! We have not evacuated. They think we have evacuated!" When nurses hear this, they try texting their friends and families that the media got it wrong. Michelle sends a cursory message to her sister Angele, telling her to call the government, CNN, anyone, and tell them they are still at the hospital. Her family hears the news report and drives to Baton Rouge, where they search the evacuation shelters for Michelle. On Wednesday night, Michelle reaches her fiance, Robert. He is shocked to hear that she never left. A shipment of supplies from the hospital's owner, UHS, is commandeered by the Federal Emergency Management Agency (FEMA).

"They were trying to get diesel in for the generator, and they couldn't get it in, there was so much red tape," explains Michelle. "I believe they made a deal. They got the diesel to Chef Highway, where there was a dry spot. They walked through the water with the big diesel barrels. They came in that way." On Wednesday, the hospital started moving patients to the hospital roof. Helicopters would be arriving. Michelle said she was "on autopilot. I just knew there was nothing I could do. There was nothing. It's not like you could do something. All I did was stay by the bedside, take care of the patients. The nurses helped move patients up flights of stairs to get them to the roof."

Sometimes it takes hours to negotiate the six flights of stairs to the roof. Bedsheets are used to move each patient, stair by stair. They try using spine boards, but they crack under the patients' weight. It is not clear if the roof can handle the weight of a helicopter, but there are no other options. Debris is removed from the roof and tossed into the water below. The first attempt by the helicopter crew to lower a personnel basket to retrieve a patient does not work.

"We didn't have many to help," Michelle says. "That was probably the worst part of the whole situation, trying to get these heavy patients upstairs and only having three nurses. We had an RT [respiratory therapist] who helped tremendously. He helped with every patient. But we didn't have anybody who wanted to help us. I know that sounds crazy. We had all of these people sitting around complaining."

They try to recruit volunteer assistance. One girl, who had to swim to the hospital, helps them. Michelle does not know her name. As they reach the top floor, they stage their patients on the floor in a conference room. They try to move one ICU patient but are unsuccessful. Plans change to evacuate the critically ill last because the move to the roof is too much for the ICU patients. There is no shelter on the roof, and oxygen tanks are running low.

On Thursday, a fleet of military helicopters arrives to assist with the evacuation. People who can walk make a human chain up the stairs to the roof. In the ICU, Michelle waits with her patients and colleagues. It is after 10:00 P.M. She feels weak. She collapses against a wall. Her colleagues place her on a bed. She awakens the next morning upset and apologizing. "I felt so bad; I was crying, saying, 'I am so sorry,' because we had people we had to take care of. I got up and I realized there were several helicopters lined up outside."

Mid-morning on Friday, September 2, 5 days after she reported to work, Michelle leaves the ICU for the last time. Before she joins others on the rooftop, the ICU staff secures medications and supplies. Soiled laundry and garbage are placed in a patient room designated as the repository for the waste.

As she waits her turn on the rooftop, employees form a buddy system. Pairs are directed by managers as to which helicopter to board. When Michelle hears one is going to Lafayette, Louisiana, she turns to her partner and says she has to leave her place. Her family is in Lafayette, and this is her helicopter. As she hears her manager yell to her not to go, Michelle turns away and jumps into the aircraft cabin. As the pilot lifts his cargo away from the hospital, Michelle looks at fires on the horizon and water everywhere. "We started crying. We were looking over and saying, 'It's gone. Total devastation. It's gone.' You could see the fire they were talking about on the radio. We flew right over Chalmette, and I am like, 'That's gone. Nothing but water. Nothing but water. Surrounded by water. Everything is gone.' It was sad. Was very sad."

They land at an airport outside of Lafayette for refueling. Michelle and two fellow nurses, including an emergency room nurse who had his wife, children, and grandmother with him, walk toward a building. Inside, men and women are on radios and phones, oblivious to the latest arrivals. They ask if they can use a phone. A woman points her finger to the right and tells them to use the pay phone.

Michelle is caught short. "'Well, we don't have any money, we just got out of the hurricane. Do you think we could use your phone?' And she kept saying, 'Pay phone is around the corner.' I said, 'Did y'all know we were coming?' She said no! Very rude. By this time, we hadn't slept. We're emotional. We lost everything. We just wanted a shower, something to eat, drink, and sleep. And our cell phones are dead. I got on the pay phone. I called collect to my aunt to get a hold of my mom, and told her, 'I am somewhere where they fuel helicopters; let everybody know and come get us.' I told her the situation of everybody else and how to get a hold of their family members. Finally, things got settled, but the shock was, 'Where are we and why won't they let us use their phone?' It was very rude. I was shocked. And they didn't care. They didn't care we were in a hurricane and at a hospital for 6 days, and just got out and were tired. They didn't care about that. They kept saying, 'Pay phone, pay phone.' We just sat there. It was tough."

Her family arrives but has to bribe someone to reach Michelle and her colleagues. Overjoyed to see them, she looks at the nurse with his family. "You should see the face on everyone—they had those dilated pupils—just drained," she says. "No smile. No frown. Just a blank stare. And since my mom and everybody were there with me, and I was the only one that had family members there," she turned to her colleague and gave her a bag. It is all that she had. "I said, 'Here, take this bag—you need this.' We called a church and they came and got that family."

Her family takes her to a nearby hotel to rest. Michelle realizes that she needs to get to a bank and cancel a check. It was for a large deposit at a French Quarter hotel where she planned to have her wedding reception. The check is the last of her savings, and she will need the money to start over. The hotel had planned to return the money as it is now occupied by FEMA workers. Safe with her family, Michelle feels angst as she watches news coverage of the devastation from Hurricane Katrina. She tells her mom she needs to go back.

"I felt like I was doing something wrong by leaving, and I needed to go back," Michelle explains. My mom, of course, the mother she is, was telling me I am doing the right thing. I am like, 'No, I'm not. They're sending nurses in. They need nurses.' When you get out you're watching the news and you're like, 'Oh, I need to go back.'"

In October, Michelle and Robert return to their flooded home. It is then that the devastation hits her. Inside her torn house are remnants from the marsh and a watermark 20 feet high. She salvages the vases that she left in the bathroom. Everything else is destroyed. On December 2, Michelle and Robert have their wedding in Norco, Louisiana. Twenty-five of their relatives and close friends attend. "My mom and sister planned my whole wedding. I would not do it. I couldn't. They kept saying, 'You're getting married.' I said, 'No, I'm not,' because all the money I had in my savings was going to go to the wedding. I needed it to start over. I can't afford flowers and a place to get married and a honeymoon and all that. And they kept saying, 'You're getting married.'"

On December 3, her sister's wedding is held at a church in the French Quarter. Following the ceremony, the sisters have a shared reception at a hall with French Quarter décor.

It matters to her to know about the experiences of other nurses who were there for the storm. "Part of healing from a traumatic experience is talking about it with your coworkers. I didn't have that," she explains. "Maybe if I read about it, it would make me feel better, because I am still extremely angry. I have so much anger about that whole situation. My husband and I don't talk about it—if we do, we get in an argument because I have so much hate about the whole situation and everything that went on. Every little step, everything that went on. If anyone says anything about Hurricane Katrina over here in Tennessee I just have to walk away because they weren't there. I have so much anger and hurt. If I read a book with other nurses in it, it would make me feel better to hear their experiences because I don't know many who went through it. Maybe I will have some peace down the road, but I don't know. Still, to this day, I don't want to hear people talking about it. They made their judgments. I had to start over from scratch. . . . It didn't have to happen, if we had evacuated from the get-go like we did with every other hurricane. If we would have evacuated, I probably wouldn't feel this angry."

And despite the trauma, Michelle says, "In a heartbeat, I would volunteer to work at a hospital facing a disaster or recovering from one.

Why? Because I have been there and I know—and I just know how to prepare. I could help in that situation."

Dionne Haun

What happened in the hospital was unbelievable. It was really a nightmare.

Dionne Haun, RN, received her BSN from the University of South Alabama, has been a registered nurse for 21 years, and has worked at Tulane University Hospital, Charity Hospital, Methodist Hospital, and St. Tammany Parish School System. Her nursing background is in labor and delivery and school nursing. Katrina was the third hurricane that she and her children had ridden out at Methodist Hospital; previously, it had been uneventful. She is married and a mother of three teenagers, plus two teenage stepchildren. Dionne recently moved to Texas and is considering starting a nurse practitioner program.

The baby could not wait. As the eye of the storm approaches New Orleans East, the labor and delivery team delivers the preemie. Mother and baby are fine—a relief to all because the power has been taken out by the hurricane-force winds and the entire hospital is relying on generator power. Dionne and her colleagues are also relieved that there would be no other patients in labor at Methodist Hospital. Those patients who were in early labor have already been transferred to a hospital out of the area. There are only four patients to take care of now. From the time she graduated from Charity School of Nursing in 1988, Dionne says she has always loved being a nurse. The fast pace and specialized area of labor and delivery attracted her. "You can't take any nurse from the hospital and tell them go induce a lady and watch that fetal pattern. We had some very good labor and delivery nurses," says Dionne.

She and the head nurse at Methodist Hospital were among the first on the nursing staff to complete fetal monitor certification courses. But on this early morning of August 29, 2005, Dionne will not need to be concerned about fetal monitoring. The eye of Hurricane Katrina has arrived, and Dionne has a front row view from the hospital's recently renovated women's unit on the third floor. A wall of glass separates her from the hurricane. Someone says the apartment complex located behind the hospital is engulfed in flames. The calm and quiet of the storm's eye belie the winds and tornadoes on its tail. The new wall of glass is solid, but Dionne can hear the crack of windows breaking in the postpartum wing. In one patient's room, a window pops near the patient's bed. "A scrub tech was helping bring some food . . . she said a window popped out spontaneously and the patient started going out with the window. They grabbed on to her leg and pulled her back. There was a lot of force when it popped out. The woman was kind of going with it," recalls Dionne.

She returns to a labor and delivery suite to check on her three children—10-year-old twin boys and a 14-year-old daughter. This is where Dionne expects they will stay for no more than 3 nights. For two previous storms, she had brought them with her to the hospital, where she had been a full-time nurse from 1989 to 2003. Now she is a school nurse in St. Tammany Parish, where she lives, but she continues working at the hospital on an as needed basis. For this storm, she expects the experience for her family will parallel those of other storms. Child care will be available as well as three meals a day. The water supply will be unlimited, and emergency generators will function until electricity returns.

"Since it had worked out so well with previous hurricanes . . . I'm thinking I will just call the hospital and see if they want me to work, because it had been always so easy to do that," she explains. "I made one phone call. Nobody really wanted to work for a hurricane. Everybody wanted to be with their family . . . and of course they wanted me there, and the kids were no problem. So that's how I got to work there.

"I just thought it was the ideal place to go for a storm. I was born and raised in St. Bernard Parish. My father was confident that where we lived in Chalmette was on very high ground. I was convinced it would never flood. The idea of anything happening like what happened for Katrina was so far out of my mind. I thought the hospital was as safe a place as it was for other storms. And the rest is history."

She and her family arrive at the hospital late Friday evening on August 26. Dionne learns that nearby Chalmette Hospital has transferred seven of their ICU patients to Methodist Hospital. On Monday, August 29, the storm passes. She is confident the worst is over. But later, the water comes. It covers parked cars and fills the hospital's first floor. Dionne's children take a bucket to retrieve water from a stairwell. The water is needed for flushing the toilet. A stop sign becomes a water gauge as employees watch the level rise.

"When the water came in, it flooded the first floor where the cafeteria, library, and morgue all went underwater. It was totally unexpected.

The generators went underwater, too. My friend's husband, who was a security officer at the hospital, swims to his truck in the parking lot. He needed a piece of equipment. He and other workers were able to get the generators working again. Then they went out and never came back on. They started plucking people off of their roofs when the emergency efforts start. . . . What happened in the hospital was unbelievable. It was really a nightmare," she says.

The storm disrupts more than human life. Flooded streets are now waterways for alligators and even a stingray. A nutria finds the top of a car the ideal place to dry off. Water seems to stretch to the horizon.

"That is all that you would see—water. And at night it was just so eerie because it was pitch black," Dionne notes. The hospital can not go on lockdown. Residents rescued from their homes keep arriving at the hospital. "We were the place. We were the only place open and everyone was coming into the hospital," says Dionne.

Among the new arrivals are a few unsavory-looking characters. Food is now in short supply. Toilets no longer flush. Employees and visitors must bag their human waste and dispose of it in a designated hallway. The stench is noxious. Hospital security venture to the adjacent Physician Plaza in search of gasoline for the generators. They return with a 92-year-old woman, whom they found in the building stairwell. No one knows where she came from because the plaza was to have been completely evacuated before the storm.

"The smell in the hospital was overwhelming," says Dionne. "People were hungry. The bottled water was beginning to run out towards the end. I don't remember running out of water as much as running out of food. The supervisor was coming around, giving us updates on what was going on. A few days after the storm someone had a radio and told us that the hospital owner was sending someone in. They were going to shrink-wrap the top of the hospital and send some kind of fumigation through it to prevent the mold from building up, because it was already starting to grow. And when we thought they weren't coming to get us, I would imagine that is pretty much when everybody started to panic."

On August 31, someone comes to the women's unit announcing that Air Force One has flown over the hospital. The hospital has a mandatory evacuation. Soon afterward, the helicopters come. As they hover around the hospital, Dionne takes photos with her cell phone. It reminds her of a war scene. Patient evacuation is under way. The first tier to leave will be ICU patients, babies, and those on the maternity floor. Visitors will leave next.

"Then there was a change in plan," offers Dionne. "We were going to send staff out before visitors and at this point it was becoming a very hostile environment at Methodist. Labor and delivery was kind of secluded and we felt that we were safe, but we thought there was going to be mutiny. The visitors were coming in. We had sterile water because we also are a surgical unit, so we could actually drink the sterile water. We were able to wash ourselves with some of these 2-L bags of fluid that we used for surgery. We felt that once they found out that we had real toilets and a little bit of food and snacks that people had brought, they were going to come into our area. It was just a matter of time.

"There were broken windows everywhere, but not in the room where we stayed. I was ready to break a window because the smell was getting so bad in there. I felt that the air was so incredibly contaminated with so many people and the human waste all over the place. It was disgusting. It was horrible smelling." She remembers the sweltering heat. "I don't know how we dealt with it, but we did."

Dionne spends the majority of her time in her unit, except when she has to go to the pharmacy. After the first floor flooded, it was relocated to the sixth floor. Dionne recalls a skeleton crew of doctors at the hospital. A new female obstetrician—gynecologist stays within the labor and delivery area. Her husband and 1-year-old child are there also. "She probably felt as I did that the hospital was the safest place to be for a hurricane," suggests Dionne.

On Friday, September 2, the labor and delivery staff is notified that it is their turn to leave. Each person can take only one small bag with her. The hospital roof has been cleared of debris. It is now a landing site. Dionne and her children join the slow procession up the stairwell. Ahead of them, an elderly female patient from the ICU is carried gingerly up the stairs by a group of nurses and volunteers. The ICU medical director stops the group to check the patient's vital signs. The physician manually suctions fluid from the woman's lungs. Dionne, 17 years a nurse, knows the sound coming from where the patient lay. One of Dionne's children turns to their mother and asks what is happening. Dionne replies softly, "She is dying. It's the death rattle."

Eventually, they reach the roof. Dionne does not know what happened to the patient. She and her children wait in line to evacuate. They are told that when they arrive at their destination, they should look for a Methodist Hospital table, where a company representative will be ready to assist. Dionne expects they will leave soon; maybe in 30 minutes. They wait for 12 hours. It is almost midnight when they board a Black Hawk helicopter. The blackness of the night envelopes the hospital campus as the helicopter lifts off from the hospital roof.

They disembark on the tarmac at Louis Armstrong International Airport. Dionne says she never feared for her life when she was at the hospital. However, as she walks with her children toward an open entry at the airport's ground level, she says, "I realized how bad a situation we were in. It was very bad." The airport baggage area is a staging area for arriving patients from evacuated hospitals and nursing homes. The scene reminds Dionne of a MASH unit. She describes it as "pitiful. My goodness, it is pitiful with all of these old people. And then if you don't need to stay down there at the makeshift hospital you were sent upstairs. I was separated from my group. We went upstairs. It was not anything I was used to being in." Dionne searches for the hospital information table. She can't find it

"At Methodist, although things are getting bad and we are out of food, I felt very comforted because I was surrounded by nurses that

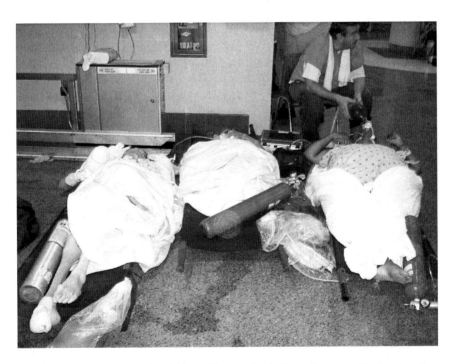

At Louis Armstrong International Airport three patients lie on the ground in the airport baggage terminal. A health care worker assists one of them. Photo by Bong Q. Mui, M.D.

I work with; some of the nurses brought their husbands, and that doctor brought her husband. It is like we are a group together and everybody is looking out for everyone. So even the visitors we thought are going to try and take over our area, we already have a plan how we are not going to let them do it. I feel protected.

"When I got to the airport I was thinking we might not make it out of here. I never thought that in the hospital. I never thought that we were going to die or anything. I was hoping the hospital wouldn't catch on fire, but when I got to that airport I got to thinking, 'Something really bad can happen and this might be the end of us.' I didn't tell that to my children, but I am just thinking, 'Someone is going to get raped, somebody is going to get kidnapped, somebody is going to get shot and killed,' because we were hearing stories of how bad the Superdome was, how bad the crime was."

Upstairs there are thousands of evacuees; many of them have spent nearly a week confined at the Superdome or the New Orleans Convention Center. There seems to be very little organization to control the crowd. Someone barks orders to get in line for buses. National Guardsmen patrol the area. They are fully armed. Dionne is not about to have her family board a bus. She fears for the safety of her children. She tells them to turn around and return downstairs. Someone calls to her, "Ma'am, once you're upstairs, you can't go back downstairs." She ignores the warning and begins walking backward down the escalator, back to the triage area in baggage. She approaches a National Guardsman, a machine gun slung over his shoulder.

"I told him I am sorry, I am not going back up there, I don't feel safe and I am really afraid someone is going to grab one of my kids. So I put my kids to sleep right under that National Guardsman. He was standing there with a machine gun. They were lying on the floor in the airport . . . it was very cold and I covered them with cardboard and tried to get them to go to sleep. And I was just about ready to attempt to go to sleep myself when I saw other people from Methodist get off, and they saw me. They said there is a place upstairs where medical people are. I said I couldn't find it. They said come on. I followed them . . . there was a place, goodness, so much better than the rest of the airport." They are given water and meals ready to eat. She manages to text her family in Shreveport to let them know where they had evacuated. They reply that her cousin, a Causeway police officer, will come to the airport and get her. Two hours later, he is there. "I don't know how in the world he found me," she says. "He was there in no time. As he came walking through the airport in his police uniform, he really stood out, it was like Jesus Christ had came down from heaven and just saved us. . . . We just walked out with him and I really felt very guilty leaving the rest of the people that I worked with there, but I really had to. I followed him, and the police car was there, and we got in. The streets were deserted. There was no one on the streets except emergency people. We were able to get on the Causeway when other people could not. . . . We went past the loop where all the people were standing on the interstate. We went straight to Mandeville . . . to my house, which had very little damage. I filled up my bathtub, didn't have hot water but that was OK . . . a bath was just phenomenal. After that I was clean, I was happy, my house was OK, and that was good."

Dionne phones her parents. While at the hospital, she had learned about the breaks in the levees and that probably most of St. Bernard Parish was underwater, yet she found the news incredulous. "You just don't believe that," she admits. "You think, 'Oh yeah, part of it is flooding,' but we had no idea of the impact of it. And then some of the people I worked with in St. Bernard Parish lived in the Lexington neighborhood and they said Lexington is completely underwater. It is completely gone. And still I just didn't believe it. They said all of Chalmette is underwater. I didn't believe it until my cousin came and picked me up . . . he had already been to Chalmette—he got on a boat . . . said, 'It's all under.' My dad's house. One of my sisters, her place was wiped out in Violet. She had about 9 feet of water. She lost that. She lost the camper, her business went under. My brother lost his house, his place of business. My other sister had a beautiful 4,000-square-foot home. She had 10 or 11 feet in that. Everyone lost everything. And that is when I really believed it."

Dionne's parents come to live with her. In 2007, they buy a house in her neighborhood. She is thrilled for them. Her mother, who had been ill, dies 6 months later. Dionne believes that the stress of her mother witnessing Dionne's sisters and brother lose their homes took a toll on her.

"I was the one that went through the storm physically. My home wasn't wiped out, but my mom. . . . She was living with us and she was trying to deal with the loss of her home plus trying to watch her kids trying to rebuild their lives with their own children."

In February 2009, Dionne and her family moved to Katy, Texas, a suburb of Houston. She has recently remarried, and her husband's company has relocated to Houston. She misses Mandeville but says Houston offers more opportunity for her children after they graduate from high school. She has plans to return to nursing. "I had no idea how much impact Katrina would have on the whole country," she offers. "I didn't realize how global it was until probably a good while after the storm. But I know that now. We talk about Katrina all the time—everyone does. It's like A.D. and B.C.—before Katrina and after Katrina."

She is hopeful that those who read about the experiences of nurses who worked at the hospitals devastated by Hurricane Katrina will have a better understanding of the challenges they faced. Without having endured nearly 6 days at the hospital, she says she would not have the feeling and memories "and the impact on my life, my children's . . . my whole family. We were all tremendously devastated." That impact extends to her children. When her sons have a class assignment to do a poster on their hero, they ask her to guess who they chose. She does not know. They show her their poster. Their hero is Dionne.

"Me? I am the hero of what?" she asks them. "They said I was their hero to them for Katrina. And then they had to present it to the class . . . they had pictures of all of the kinds of things that happened. . . . They had this beautiful model that was me they put as a picture. . . . They said that the whole class was in awe when they told the story. And their teacher said is that really true? They said it was absolutely. . . . They got an A on it. They didn't bring the poster home yet—they said it's hanging up on the wall; everyone's is hanging on the wall, but I am really anxious to get it back because I am trying to keep all of the things from Katrina."

Sue Jester

My philosophy has always been that God takes care of fools and little children. We were the fools and we had the little children.

Sue Jester, RN, BSN, has been a RN for 26 years. She graduated from LSU School of Nursing in 1982. She has practiced nursing in the New Orleans area for most of those years. Since Hurricane Katrina, she is working on the North Shore, where she lives with her husband of 19 years and her two teenage sons.

The week before Hurricane Katrina came ashore in southeast Louisiana, Sue Jester had her hands full as night shift assistant head nurse in the nursery at Methodist Hospital. Since graduating in 1982 from LSU School of Nursing, Sue has worked in New Orleans East at Lakeland Medical Center and Methodist Hospital. Her 60-hour week has been punctuated by an increased number of births. She has not kept up with the storm's tracking. But that Sunday, August 28, when New Orleans mayor C. Ray Nagin issues a mandatory evacuation for the city, she hurries her husband, Larry, and their 12- and 10-year-old sons to pack their bags and leave their home in Slidell. They are out the door by 9:00 A.M., headed to Pensacola, where they will stay at the home of Sue's sister-in-law.

"I grew up in New Orleans, and stayed through Hurricane Betsy when I was 5," she says. "Mom was pregnant and Dad was a fireman. Only when it got to a Category 4 and 5 did we evacuate. We rode out the storm in our house in Orleans Parish. The waters came to the front door. For Hurricane Katrina, I had less than 12 hours to get my family out. My youngest son is an artist and he wanted his pictures. I told him, 'You don't have time.' They left. That was the best decision I ever made."

When she reports to work at 11:00 A.M., she anticipates that her first task will be to help patients transfer to other hospitals. Then she will leave and reunite with her family in Florida. An ambulance is transferring two babies from the neonatal ICU as she walks toward the hospital entrance. One is going to Children's Hospital in the University section of town, the other to University Hospital downtown. Since Methodist Hospital does not have a Level III Neonatal Intensive Care Nursery, Sue says regardless if there was a storm or not, these transfers would be necessary. She talks briefly to the ambulance driver. He tells her the traffic is a mess on the interstate as thousands of people are still evacuating.

The hospital nursery, located on the third floor, is quiet. Sue sees Colleen, the day shift charge nurse. They are the only two who have reported to work. Their director is on vacation. About five o'clock, Sue and Colleen are still hoping other nurses will report to work. They are told by their supervisor that it will be the two of them for the storm. An obstetrician, is on the labor and delivery unit. With her are her husband and toddler.

"My philosophy has always been that God takes care of fools and little children. We were the fools and we had the little children," she smiles. "And we knew that we could depend on each other. If something was bad we could wake each other up."

Their patients are two NICU babies less than 1 day old. The medical staff have advised the new mothers not to evacuate with the newborns. It is best for the babies that they remain at the hospital. The mother of one has evacuated to the Superdome. The other mother is headed to Houston. A third patient is in the well-baby nursery whose mother has stayed at the hospital.

"We all thought the safest place would be at the hospital," observes Sue, "but the storm and its aftermath were an eye-opener for all of us."

The nursery is a secured area located in the back of the recently renovated women's floor. One large picture window allows daylight to flood the area. Sunday night is quiet for Sue. She fills all the open containers she can find with water. It is something she always does for major storms. The water reserves may be needed. When the hurricane approaches, she expects more, but there is "a dead calm. It was truly the calm before the storm," she says softly.

She works through early morning. In the background, she can hear the recording by Michael Bublé—"I Want to Go Home." She calls it their theme song. When Colleen reports, she tells Sue to get breakfast. The cafeteria on the first floor is jammed with people—families, National Guard, policemen. It is raining, but not hard. When she returns to the unit, she locates an empty patient room to share with a postpartum nurse who works the day shift.

"All of a sudden, I hear screaming. It is almost 9:30 A.M. The windows are blowing out. As I walk to the far end of the floor, I hear a weird noise. I open the door to a patient room. Inside there is a patient, probably moved from the medical/surgical unit. Ceiling tiles are on top of him. We move the patient. I told the security guy this is why we should evacuate. People are screaming we are going to blow away. I tell them the hospital's safe. More windows blow out on the third floor. That's when I really got nervous. I didn't think it was a tornado, and with the window open, it was the force of the wind. I had gone down earlier to the lobby, when the pressure was changing. You couldn't even walk to the door [there] because there was so much pressure. That's when the trees were bending. There was a National Guard truck outside and it seemed like the wind would push the truck through the windows. That's when I called my family and said, 'I don't know if we're going to make it.' I talked with my husband. My sister-in-law had ridden out Hurricane Ivan in a closet at her home. She said I know what you're going through. It's going to be over. I told her, 'It's never going to be over.'" Her voice falters. "We cried, and I told them I loved them. That was hard."

From the nursery, Sue and Colleen can see the apartment complex behind the hospital. There is an explosion. The building is soon engulfed in flames. Other fires can be seen in the distance. Knowing that there are only a few hours before she starts the night shift, Sue tries to rest. She has been awake since 5:00 A.M. Sunday. "I lie down. It is now 10 o'clock. That is when the water comes. It was like a wave came through, with whitecaps. The first floor is underwater. I am thinking we are going to die."

Employees race to salvage what they can from the first floor as the water rises to the ceiling. Sue calls it "surreal. You don't know what to think. As far as emotions I guess it's like a death. You are thinking, how are we getting out of here? Someone says the interstate is clear. We talk about swimming to higher ground. If we can get to the interstate, we're going to walk home. I did not know there were no twin spans." (The Interstate 10 Twin Span Bridge is composed of 5.4-mile-long parallel bridges that span the eastern end of Lake Pontchartrain from New Orleans to Slidell.) Storm surge has caused extensive damage to the bridges and shifted some segments off their piers.

When she surveys the neighborhood from the third floor, Sue sees stingrays and turtles in the waters below. Soon raw sewerage and oil from the drowned cars will ooze into the waters. Maybe swimming is not the way to leave. A man marooned in a tree above the rising water screams for help. Some hospital employees shout back, "Swim to us."

At 2:00 P.M., Sue hears that the hospital owner, UHS, is sending supplies. Four hours later, the hospital CEO announces that the shipment has been commandeered. They will not be getting anything. Soon the hospital will be losing power. There is another delivery in labor and delivery. The baby is fine. Night descends, and Sue hopes for another quiet shift. The air-conditioning went out hours ago. The humidity is high and the heat is heavy. A surveillance plane is heard passing over the hospital. It shines a light on the marooned building. Someone suggests that they make an SOS sign, but the plane is gone, leaving the blackness of the night.

News filters to Sue and Colleen through one of the obstetrician techs, whose husband works in hospital maintenance. The best place to get cell phone satellite reception is on the fourth-floor observation deck. Sue reaches her husband. She tells him they are flooded, but OK. On Monday night, volunteers are needed to help hand-bag the ventilator-dependent patients in the ICU. The police and National Guardsmen assist. Sue is grateful that the night shift stay is uneventful, except for the fact the hospital is now an island.

On Tuesday, an intensive care nurse goes into labor. She is airlifted from Methodist. Sue is hopeful that the babies will be next. Later that day, a woman in labor comes to the hospital by boat. Her family had tried to transport her in an open refrigerator, but when it sank, a boater came to their rescue. The boat docks outside the second floor of the hospital.

The woman is carefully lifted through a broken window. Sue says the interior of the building "is starting to sweat." The staff is concerned if a cesarean section will be needed. Moisture has compromised the surgical suite. Fortunately, there is no surgery, and the preterm baby is fine. The nursery now has five babies.

Medications are replenished at the pharmacy, which was moved from the first floor to the sixth. For one of the babies, there is no more of a necessary medication.

"It was caffeine. We tried to figure out how much caffeine was in a can of Coke, how much to give the baby," explains Sue. "We would have to give an ounce, but we thought the baby would throw it up because it is a carbonated beverage. Then we decided the baby, who was not severely preterm, could be watched by us because we had no electricity for the monitor. As long as someone kept their eyes on him, or kept him close to their chest, we would know if he went into distress.

"It was hot that night," she continues. "We had the two NI [neonatal intensive] babies crying because the temperature was so high. My little pans of water came in handy. I was able to sponge them down. None of them got a heat diaper rash. I am very proud of that."

The darkness in the hospital is stark. An elderly man who has found refuge on the third floor tells Sue he lost everything in Hurricane Betsy. He doesn't think he can do it again with Katrina. Sue assures him that they are going to make it through.

While she watches her small patients, Sue assures herself that rescue will soon come. Surely the plane that flew over them Monday night has reported signs of life at the hospital. An emergency radio is tuned to station WWL. People are calling with their eyewitness reports. The Slidell community of Eden Isles by Lake Pontchartrain is gone. That means Colleen has lost everything. A woman calls to say she can drive along Gauze Boulevard, a thoroughfare in Slidell. South of the city is underwater. That means the home of Sue's mother-in-law is flooded.

"I didn't think there was anything left of our home, but my family was safe. We'll just start over," Sue says.

Sue sleeps 3 hours at most, "just to get the exhaustion out." On Tuesday, she camps out in an operating room where it is cooler, dark, and away from noise. Elsewhere on the unit, some families watch a movie on a battery-powered DVD player. Sue says everyone was in "survival mode. Everybody was doing their best. Whatever we had, we shared with them."

Because of the heat, Sue is not hungry, but she makes herself eat half a sandwich. She needs to maintain her stamina and watch her high blood pressure. The discovery of a frozen liter of Coke in the back of the unit freezer is welcome. The semithawed brown liquid is shared among the group. Sue takes a swallow, and there is a burning sensation in her throat. It does not matter. The liquid is cold. She checks on supplies. There are plenty of ready-to-feed formulas. However, later that Tuesday, someone raids the nursery and takes the gift packets and some formula.

"We don't know how, or who let them in. Our nursery is locked. Colleen and the nurses from labor and delivery got the rest of the formula that we felt we needed and put it in carts by labor and delivery."

On Wednesday, the National Guard and police leave the hospital to join in search and rescue. Some people become anxious as they leave. Others get restless. Sue hears later that some of those who found refuge at the hospital threatened to kill the employees if they are not rescued first. "They thought they were going to take the staff and leave everybody else," Sue recounts. "The administrators told them, 'If you start killing us, they're leaving and they're not coming back for you.' That's how they got everybody calm again."

For rest, Sue lies on a pallet placed on the nursery floor. Sue feels her lowest that day. She prays the rosary, and when she starts her shift, there is good news. The babies and moms will be evacuated. She and a labor and delivery nurse will go with them. They are instructed to take only one bag. Sue crams formulas and diapers in her lab coat pockets. Colleen and Sue discharge their patients and give each mom her discharge instructions. The nurses stop charting. Sue takes baby Zachary and begins her ascent with the others up four flights of stairs to the roof. She holds Zachary close to her chest. The labor and delivery nurse does the same with her tiny charge. Sue feels the effects of her hypertension. She is dizzy. She knows that she is dehydrated. They make it to the roof. The heat is oppressive. They wait with the five moms, and four of them cradle their newborns. An hour passes. At three o'clock, they are instructed to return to the third floor. It is unsafe for a helicopter to land because of the loose gravel that covers the roof.

They return to the third floor, dejection on their faces. They quietly unload their bags. The doctor's husband surveys the group and announces that he is taking them out to dinner. They can order anything on the menu. What would you like? Sue pipes up, "A margarita! And ice!" The others join in. Their virtual dining experience seems to lift their spirits.

At 6:00 P.M., a runner brings word that they are going to try the evacuation again. They fortify themselves with bites from a sandwich. They wait for an hour on the roof, and then the evacuation is called off because it is getting dark. They return to the third floor. All are exhausted. They decide not to listen to the radio. At 10:15, Sue borrows a cell phone and calls her husband. She tells him about the failed rescue. She asks, "Is the family OK?" They are. She tells him they plan to evacuate tomorrow and that she will call when she reaches her destination, but no one knows where that will be. The mothers retire to their rooms with their babies. Sue fights fatigue and places a chair between the two cribs that hold her patients. She sits in the chair and rests her arm next to each baby. What seems like a few minutes pass, when Sue is startled by another runner. They need to go back to the roof. Her first reaction is that they cannot go. Everyone has retired, but the labor and delivery nurse readies moms with their babies. As Colleen stuffs medical charts in her bag, Sue crams formula and diapers in her pockets. Sue pulls her lab coat over her pajamas and puts her shoes on her sockless feet. For the third time, the group makes their way to the roof, where a Black Hawk helicopter hovers. For previous rescue attempts, ropes have been thrown from the helicopter's open side. Sue cannot imagine being lifted to the helicopter while holding her tiny patient. The plan to pull evacuees up is halted. The ropes are released and the helicopter lands.

It is 11:00 P.M. Those who are waiting to leave are draped with a sheet to help shield them from any flying debris caused by the rotating helicopter blades. Colleen calls her sister in California. She gives her the phone number of Zachary's mom and asks her to notify her that they are evacuating. They will call again when they arrive at their destination. As they wait on the roof, the chief nursing officer hands them a piece of paper with UHS information and an 800 number to call.

"They handed us a paper that stated we'll rehire you when the hospital opens. You're like, my God. I have the babies, I have no job. I had some choice words in my head, but by that time I am just get me out of here. We'll do the details later."

A labor and delivery nurse is to evacuate with them. However, she is missing. Sue, Colleen, and two of the moms are motioned to board the helicopter. On board is a patient from the women's unit. Sue is handed the patient's chart.

"They handed us her chart and said, 'Take care of her like you would our babies,'" says Sue. "We climb in and sit on the floor. Our legs are cramping, but I am smiling. We are leaving."

When their helicopter lands, Sue says the darkness makes it difficult to see where they are. As they disembark, they profusely thank the flight crew. The helicopter lifts off and the charts in Colleen's bag fly out. She and Sue chase them. Sue turns and sees a sign. It reads "Causeway Boulevard." "Why are we here?" Her vision adjusts to the darkness. What she sees reminds her of a post–Mardi Gras parade route. There seems to be thousands of people. Litter is everywhere. They see a police officer and ask, where do they go? They have babies and new moms. They can't stay there. He points to the underpass, where they find another policeman. They are told an ambulance will arrive. They see a resident, an orthopedist from Charity Hospital.

"He says he is trying to help as best he could," says Sue. "He gives us a bottle of water. It was hot. I think, 'What happened? There is no ice in the world? This is New Orleans in August, when it is 90° at night and there is 100% humidity. Everybody here is going to die.' There were old, frail people. Then around 11:00 P.M., it must have been God helping us, we see the other two moms getting on an ambulance. We run to them. We are back together again."

As the ambulance leaves, Sue asks where they are going. There is no reply. They are brought to Louis Armstrong International Airport. As they walk through the ground-level baggage area, the floor space is covered by elderly patients lying on mats. It is Thursday, September 1, 1:00 A.M., when Sue and Colleen, each holding a baby, followed by the mothers, are in line for processing. They give their names and what hospital they came from. No one asks how they are. There is no triage for them.

"This is the first time in the world anybody asks our name, because until then, I don't think UHS knew I was there, since all the time clocks went underwater," offers Sue. "I don't think they are that impersonal, but I don't think anyone ever took a list of who had been at the hospital. Maybe they did know, but from my perspective I don't think anybody knew where I was or what happened to the babies."

They are directed to the second floor, where a field hospital is set up at the west end of the concourse.

"Anyone who would listen, I told them that we have babies we have to get out of here. And it wasn't a selfish thing. I wanted these babies out of there. They were newborns! And it looked like nursing home patients all around there. I try to find out who is in charge. Finally, there is a woman who tells me we will be among the first ones to leave in the morning. We found a little place away from everybody, dark, where the moms and babies—we were across from the bathroom. They had water

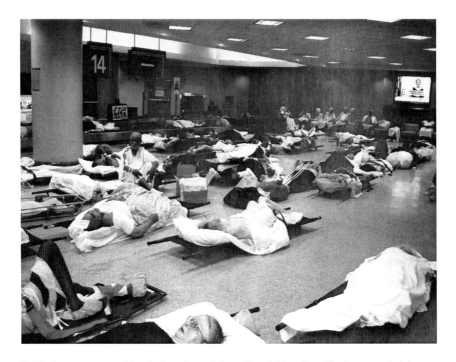

In the baggage area of Louis Armstrong International Airport, patients evacuated from flooded hospitals and nursing homes lie on the floor awaiting evacuation from New Orleans. Photo by Bong Q. Mui, M.D.

so we could wash. The water wasn't cold, but it wasn't hot. There are large tubes that pump cool air inside."

Once the moms and babies are settled, Sue leaves to scout out the area and find a soft-drink machine. There is none. Her group has not eaten. No one offers them any food. A man approaches them. He says he can take them to Baton Rouge. Sue tells the mothers she does not trust the stranger. She says they are not under her care anymore but believes it is best if they stay together. The man loans them his cell phone. The moms call their families. The man tells them a plane has left. Sue seeks out the woman she talked with earlier. When she finds her, the woman tells Sue not to bother her.

Undaunted, Sue searches for someone who can help. By 10:00 A.M., they board a tram that will take them across the tarmac to a military plane. The sun is beating down as they sit in this tram. Sue tells the moms that the babies are getting hot. They need to go back inside. She sees someone who has orange juice and asks if she can get some for the moms because it has been several hours since all of them last ate. Each has only one warm water bottle kept in their pockets. They get some juice.

Another plane is scheduled to leave at noon. Sue and the others are in the first group. They line up again. If their name is not on the list, they will not be able to get on the buses. Someone comes up to Sue and asks if he can sneak into the line. Sue tells the stranger to back off. She is not breaking up her group. As they walk to the buses, CNN interviews the moms about their ordeal. Sue's friends recognize her and call her later. Finally, all of them board the C130. They sit in the jump seats. In the middle section of the plane are patients lying on stretchers. Sue holds baby Zachary close to her.

"We are told they were going to feed us," says Sue. "Then somebody went into cardiac arrest and they had to resuscitate them. So we never got anything to eat. I sat down and dozed off. When I awoke, I told the moms to wake up their babies and make them cry to help alleviate pressure in their ears. I look down at Zachary. I pat him and he smiles. It was like he was saying, 'Oh, I finally got out of there. Everything is going to be all right now.' He just smiled. He would never cry."

The plane lands in Fort Worth. A media frenzy greets the arriving evacuees. Cameras flash.

"We don't have any press releases for these babies," protests Sue. "I am still in hospital mode. A guy pulls up with a wheelchair. I tell him, 'I am not a patient. I am a nurse.' He says, 'You have to sit down, ma'am.' I tell him again, 'I am a nurse. I have got the patient.' He says, 'Regulations, ma'am.' 'Well,' I think, 'somebody's in charge.'"

The neonatal intensive babies are directed to Cook Children's Hospital. The others and their moms will be brought to another hospital. Sue and Colleen give their reports on each baby and the patient charts. They also give the staff their moms' contact numbers. Colleen calls her sister again to tell her they have landed in Fort Worth and to call Zachary's mother with the Fort Worth phone number.

"One of the nurses asks us, 'What are we going to do?' Colleen and I look at each other. We didn't think the whole time what we are going to do," admits Sue. "It's like we are abandoned. The nurse says she is from the NICU. 'Do we want to ride with the transport team?' We say, 'OK.' She goes to take the babies from our arms. We had the babies in our arms for 14 hours and it was hard to let go. Finally, when she took the baby, it was like this big relief.

"This is Thursday, September 1. It's a new month. It's a new world. As they put one of the babies in the ambulance, Colleen and I look at each other. What do we do now? You are still in survival mode because you are in a strange place. I am here alone, no money, no identity, and no job. But I knew that my family was safe. I have $60 in my purse and a credit card. I don't know if it works. How are we getting home? We have no car. We have nothing. I tell Colleen, 'We are in Texas; we'll have to first have some Mexican food and then we'll figure out the rest.'"

At the hospital, they meet the nurse director of the neonatal intensive care unit. Sue calls her a godsend. She asks how they are, what they need. They are brought to the physicians' lounge, where they shower and change into fresh scrubs. There is a phone they can use to call anyone they need to reach. The director and her husband take them out for a Mexican meal. Before they leave, they stop by the nursery to check on the babies. All are fine.

Colleen makes contact with her son, who evacuated to Denton, located north of Dallas. Sue decides to stay in Fort Worth so she can be close to the airport. She spends the night at the director's home. Sleep comes easily for her. The following morning, she is told that Zachary's family is on the *Good Morning America* television program. They are telling his story and how the nurses got him safely to Texas.

Sue does not know the status of her home. She calls the 800 number on her sheet of paper. She asks if they rescued the labor and delivery staff. She is told there is no information on that. She asks if they will arrange for her travel home. She had gone on a patient transfer for them. She has no credit cards that work. Can they help her get home? Again, there is no information. As the director's husband works for Southwest Airlines, he helps arrange a direct flight to connect her with her family in Pensacola.

Sue returns to the hospital, where the director gives her a tour of the women's unit. "She says, 'If you don't have a job, come here.' I did apply later," Sue says. "I went there to find a house, check my kids into school, and things didn't fall into place. The house fell through and I was going to get an apartment and commute. But then I found a job near home." Waiting for her flight, Sue sits by the assigned gate. Inside her lab coat pocket, she fingers her Methodist Hospital badge. She stares at the television, which is streaming reports about Hurricane Katrina's devastation. She starts crying.

"I still wasn't feeling anything. I didn't know why I was crying. I know now. But at that time, I was going through the motions, and inside, I couldn't feel it. People were trying to console me. One of them was a nurse returning to California. She told me to come to California. She would give me a job.

"Once we are in flight, I looked out and could see the Mississippi Gulf Coast line. It was wiped out. There was nothing on the beaches. When I get to Florida, my sons are there with flowers and balloons. My husband and his brother had gone to Slidell to check on our home. My sons tell me I look puny. They took me to eat. Everybody wants to feed you."

Sue believes the hurricane and hospital evacuation took its toll on many people. In September, she has an outbreak of shingles and is later diagnosed with diabetes. She keeps in contact with her former colleagues from Lakeland and Methodist, many of whom were her coworkers those 20 years.

"They were there at my wedding and for my children's births. I had been at theirs. We knew each other when we dated our husbands. We had been through so much together. Illnesses. Celebrations. We were like a family. For me, I don't think I lost it all, but I definitely miss the people. We still get together whenever possible."

Reflecting on those 4 days at Methodist, Sue says she felt that she was with family. "Even though you did kind of feel alone, you felt like you had somebody else watching your back. You're in the survival mode. This is kind of like your family. If this is the end of the world, these are the people you want to be with. I think that's why the mothers, the babies, Colleen . . . we all had this trust. We were all we had."

When a relative suggests that Sue needs to have therapy, she responds that she doesn't have the time. "I think we had therapy at work," she offers. "If you had tough times, you talked about it, we cried, we laughed. At the year anniversary, we were going to do a come-as-you-were-for-Katrina party, but because it was still so raw at 1 year and the memories were harder, we thought, 'Maybe we will do it at the 10-year mark.'"

In October 2005, after the storm, Sue returns to Methodist to collect her personal items. The hospital is a shell. The interior has been stripped.

"When I went back, that was the hardest thing. I went alone. They had security. A guide went with me to my office that I had shared with Colleen. Plastic was everywhere. I gathered my pillows and belongings I had left. I cried. As I was leaving, a man came up to me and tried to console me. He said, 'I know this is hard for you.'"

Also in October, Sue accepts a job at a hospital near her home. When Hurricane Gustav made landfall west of Grand Isle, Louisiana, on September 1, 2008, Sue was working. Any trepidation she had about this hurricane was calmed by her colleagues, several of whom had been at Methodist for Hurricane Katrina.

"So many people believe that Katrina just happened to New Orleans," she says. "They don't think that it can happen anywhere else. Even the Mississippi Gulf Coast was totally wiped out. What I took from this experience is that you cannot depend on anyone else taking care of you. You have got to stand up and take care of yourself and be prepared. Always have your nursing license and three sets of scrubs with you. Never be without two or three cases of water. Always be prepared."

She adds that disasters mean "you never stop nursing because that's what we do. Patients are like your family. You would take care of your family and you would definitely take care of your patients. Getting those babies out of there, I knew we could do it. I was worried because they were so little and were being subjected to everything. . . . Hopefully there will be policy changes. I know that nurses will be prepared and they can make a difference. They can do anything. I feel that we just survived from one minute to the next. It wasn't just me. It was every nurse there."

6   Chalmette Medical Center

Chalmette Medical Center opened in 1977 as a 109-bed acute care facility located in St. Bernard, Louisiana, and functioned in that capacity for 25 years. In February 1981, De La Ronde Hospital opened across the street, with 118 beds. The two hospitals were consolidated into one medical center (St. Bernard Parish, 1999). Universal Health Services acquired Chalmette Medical Center, then a 196-bed acute care hospital, in 1983. The hospital served the residents of St. Bernard Parish; many of the hospital employees' families had lived in that neighborhood and grown up there for generations.

The hospital had just completed a $17 million wing before Hurricane Katrina. Chalmette Medical Center was decimated by Katrina and the subsequent levee failure that flooded the hospital and surrounding area with at least 12 feet of water. Included in the hospital's property was an adjacent 47,000-square-foot medical office building and a physical rehabilitation skilled nursing facility, which was finally demolished in 2007 (Bazile, 2007).

In 2005, after Hurricane Katrina, the primary medical services for St. Bernard residents were provided in a clinic set up in a vacant Walmart parking lot. Currently health care services are provided in a 22,000-square-foot mobile unit funded by the Franciscan Mission of Our Lady of the Lake Health System out of Baton Rouge.

Five nurses recount their stories of courage, bravery, and dedication to their patients and the profession of nursing, which they so proudly displayed at Chalmette Medical Center during and after the catastrophic storm.

Rae Ann Deroché

There's no air, the window is open. It's just still. You don't hear the birds. You hear people screaming for help. You hear a child crying, "Help me, help me." And what could we do? You could hear boats every now and then and the screams would get so loud. It was a nightmare.

Rae Ann Deroché, RN, was born and raised in St. Bernard Parish, where she met her spouse, Daryl, and was raising her family. Rae Ann started as a nursing aide at the original Chalmette General Hospital and remained there over the years as it changed owners. The hospital was her other home where she cared for the people in her community. She calls it a wonderful place for her to work because she took care of the people in her community. Rae Ann graduated from Charity School of Nursing in New Orleans in 1984.

"This is my community, this is where I was born and raised," she explains. "Everybody I took care of was somebody's momma that I grew up with. I was taking care of friends, family, or cousins of friends or family. It was just a small community out here. I took care of the people I knew."

She had been at the hospital when Hurricane Georges prompted a mandatory evacuation order for New Orleans in September 1998, and she was there for Hurricane Ivan in 2004. Both storms jogged away from New Orleans. Ivan devastated Pensacola, Florida. So on that last Friday in August 2005, she calls work to check on her schedule as a charge nurse on a telemetry unit. She works 12-hour shifts Monday, Tuesday, and Wednesday. When Rae Ann inquires what preparations are under way, she is told, "We're sitting tight."

On Saturday, watching the news coverage on Hurricane Katrina, Rae Ann knows "it was going to get ugly." She sends her 18-year-old daughter and two sons, ages 16 and 10, to Southeastern University in Hammond, Louisiana, where her daughter is 2 weeks into her freshman year. Her husband, Daryl, has recently received notice that pink slips are imminent for his job with the New Orleans school system. He tells her that if she has to stay for the storm, he will, too.

"I knew if I didn't go in to work, I didn't have a job. Both of us can't lose a job at the same time," she explains. One of her sisters tells her she and her family are evacuating to Baton Rouge. Rae Ann asks her to take her three children with her.

"We were going to get hit. We are going to get it and I had never been afraid before, but I was this time. I knew it was going to be bad. I called Saturday after I sent my children off. I spoke to the supervisor. I asked, 'Are we evacuating?' She said, 'No, we're not.' That was about three o'clock. I called back about six. 'Have we started evacuating yet?' I ask. She said, 'No, Rae Ann, we are not evacuating. Don't call me again.' I waited 'til nine o'clock, when the other nurse supervisor was on. I called him and asked, 'Have you started moving patients out yet?' He said, 'No, we haven't moved anybody. We are just sitting tight.' I am thinking, 'What the hell is wrong with you people?' I am a staff nurse who is asking, why aren't these people out yet? What do you have going on? What are the plans?"

Although she was not privy to administration's storm planning, she was stunned that there would be no early evacuation. "I don't care how you look at it, it was a major administrative screw-up. They could not see what was heading their way. Anything Category 4 coming close, you know the thing's got a wide berth. Come on, guys. Get the hell out of town! It was coming! Direct hit or not, we were still going to get it. Let's face it. We're a two-story hospital. All of our electronics are on the first floor. ICU [the intensive care unit] is on the first floor. Generators and lab. The only thing that was upstairs are patients and nursing offices."

On Sunday, August 28, Rae Ann and Daryl board up their house in Violet, a subdivision a few miles south of the hospital. They head to the home of her mother-in-law, who lives in Arabi, adjacent to Chalmette, where they shutter that home. The winds are increasing. It is nearing 2:00 P.M. when they drive to the hospital.

Chalmette Medical Center has 54 patients that cannot be discharged. Earlier, patients in the ICU had been transferred to Methodist, Chalmette's sister hospital. Most of the patients had been evacuated. An additional seven patients are admitted the night of the storm. Rae Ann says that at Chalmette Medical Center, people were dropping off family members at the emergency room (ER) and leaving. She had seen it before for other storms.

"The one I really felt sorry for was an elderly man who brought his wife who had lung cancer. She was on oxygen. He came to the hospital and said, 'I don't want to stay at home alone with her.' What do you say?

He is in his 80s, his wife is dying of lung cancer, she needs her pain medicine, and I understand all of this. He couldn't evacuate her, but where's family? I guess I was raised with a large family that I could depend upon. Not everybody is that fortunate. He came to us. That is about the only one I understood. The rest were just dropping them off and taking off because they didn't want to be bothered."

As the storm nears landfall, Rae Ann focuses on her patients. The hurricane makes its course across the southeastern part of the state. Rae Ann feels they have weathered the storm better than she had thought they would. She heads to the medicine room—she needs to get medication for one of her patients. A large window offers a view of the rear parking lot. Finishing her task, Rae Ann suddenly notices a movement in the distance. It is coming toward her.

"I see this thing rolling. I look. You do a double take, and just like you see the water rolling up on a beach. It just kept rolling," she says. "It just never stopped. It went across the parking lot and I saw it hit the wall. Then it just kept going."

She raises her hands up above her head. "Then you saw it rise. As I saw it rolling across the packed parking lot, I don't know what expletive I used, but I said something, and 'Get in here!' People came running in and there's the water just rolling through. My sister-in-law Cindy calls me and says, 'Rae Ann, I just heard the levee broke.' I said, 'Well, I see the water.' I said, 'I'll let you know how we do.' And I hung up with her. She was in Baton Rouge and heard on the radio all that nightmare stuff. They were trying to find out anything they could about us."

Racing against time, employees pull extra food and medicine and anything they think will be useful. They stack containers with food. Pharmacy quickly relocates to the administration office area. Patients are moved to one wing. The remaining wings are used to house supplies and employees. Several staff members had their families with them. Ages ranged from infants to the elderly.

By noon, the rolling waters are now 8 feet deep. Rae Ann and her colleagues use the nursing home located behind the hospital as a water gauge. She turns to a physician and asks him how much longer it will be before the water stops rising. He estimates another 4 hours.

"Eight feet in 4 hours," Rae Ann calculates. "So 8 feet from eight o'clock to noon. Noon to four, we are talking 15, 20 feet of water. I figured if this water keeps coming in, we're not going to make it. This is it!

"I had been strong because we had a bunch of young nurses and their fiancés and husbands and I was, quote, unquote, who they called

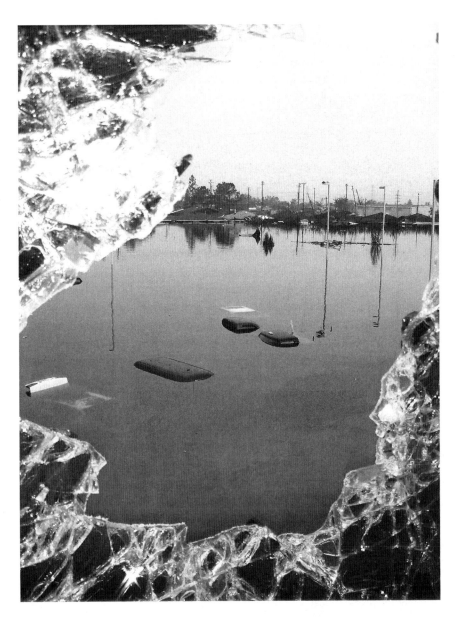

A broken second-floor window at Chalmette Medical Center frames the view of submerged cars in the parking lot. Photo by Bong Q. Mui, M.D.

'Momma Nurse.' I was one of the older nurses who worked the floor. My nickname was 'Momma Nurse' because I told them I could have given birth to any one of them. So I was trying to be the strong one for them. When he told me that, I went inside the medicine room, sat down, and cried because I figured that was it. That there is no way we're going to make it out. Who do you pull to the roof?

"Survival was starting to come through. 'Oh, my God, what do I do? If we all get on the roof, it's gonna go' . . . all of these thoughts were going through my head. I am thinking, 'I am not strong enough to swim to survive' . . . that's when I just lost it."

The husband of one of the nurses sees Rae Ann in the medicine room. He leaves to find her husband. Daryl comes and tells her they will be all right. They have boats.

"I guess he was trying to make me feel better, but when you think about it logistically, the number of people and the six or so boats didn't add up. He was coaxing me to get strong again. I went back to taking care of my patients. I had one woman tell me she was so ticked off because she can't believe we can't get an electrician to fix the air-conditioner. I told her, 'Ma'am, there is about 8 feet of water outside. I don't think any electrician wants to work in that water.' She said, 'We got water?' I nodded my head."

Family members of patients had not brought their own food supplies. Many left their personal medications in their cars, which are now underwater. The first floor floods; electricity, water, and phones are cut off.

"Here we are trying to get doctors to write prescriptions because you have a person with high blood pressure and heart disease who needs his pills. You weren't just treating the patients. You were treating family members. You had to treat them. You could not not treat them. The doctor is giving a mini–patient interview to find out what's wrong with them, writing prescriptions so that we can go get medicine for them. It was a nightmare," says Rae Ann.

When the electricity goes out, the nursing staff know the pumps will last 2 hours on battery. When a pump stops for a patient on a cardiac drip, the nurses start manually regulating the pump.

Relates Rae Ann, "You are there calculating . . . counting drops. We watch her throughout the entire shift. Then the medicine runs out. She starts going into distress. We call the doctor. We are out of this medicine, what do we want to try? I said, 'Get a pharmacist in here because they know what they have. I can't tell you.' So we have a doctor at the bedside, a pharmacist at the bedside, and the nurse. We are trying to figure out what can we set up to give this patient because she is going into distress. We were just trying everything."

Rae Ann says that even the process of getting medications became labor-intensive. Nurses could no longer access the medications. They stood in line at the relocated pharmacy.

"But we had over 50 patients that needed medicine," she says. "So here you are, you have a line that took 2 or 3 hours to get medicine. The Pyxis machines didn't work without electricity. The pharmacist had to go through a paper schematic of the drugs located in the machine, and then manually open the drawer to retrieve the medicine."

While she is on her shift, Daryl is busy helping with various tasks. When the kitchen floods, the staff use a grill that Daryl fashions out of grates from a linen cart. He connects a propane tank to the creation; they use it to grill chicken. A roof vent is cleaned and used as a pot.

"My husband helped us a lot," says Rae Ann. "I was telling my mom the other day, I was so mad at him for not taking care of my children. I said this is my responsibility. You need to go with the children. But had he not gone with me, I wonder how much worse off we would have been, because he did so much for us."

Rae Ann does not listen to the radio "because I felt like I was dealing with too much. I didn't want to deal with more bad news. People were coming in and telling you, 'Did you hear this?' I needed to focus. I didn't want to lose myself again."

When her shift ends, Rae Ann stays on the floor, "trying to help the ones that are coming on behind you, because you already know what a nightmare it is because you were in it. You are trying to help them get organized, mentally and emotionally prepared for their shift." She leaves her unit and heads toward the roof to join Daryl. One of the orderlies calls out to her for assistance. She helps him. She heads to the stairs. Another call for Rae Ann. Someone is having chest pains.

"I turned around and said, 'Get the nurse on duty. I'm done!' I kept walking. And that's not like me to turn my back, but I couldn't go any more. I had to get out. After 12–14 grueling hours, I was done. I went up to the roof and my husband was there. Everybody was trying to use phones. A few people could text. Every now and then, we'd get a text message. I did not know how to text. Neither did my husband, but we are now technologically advanced. We know this. A phone was a phone then, but now it is so much more."

About 11:00 p.m., she and Daryl try to rest on the second floor. "There's no air, the window is open. It's just still. You don't hear the birds. You hear people screaming for help. You hear a child crying help me, help me. And what could we do? You could hear boats every now and then and the screams would get so loud. It was a nightmare," she says. Some of the men in the hospital have taken their boats to bring stranded people to the hospital for shelter. An estimated additional 400 storm survivors are now in the hospital. The parish jail and the area around Paris Road are dry. A physician scouts out the jail and deems it a good place to set up a mini-MASH unit. Jail cells are converted to hospital rooms. On Tuesday, August 30, the hospital staff start transporting patients to the jail, in addition to medical staff and supplies. For every six patients that are transferred, a nurse accompanies them. Patients' medications are placed in plastic bags and put inside their charts.

"If the patient couldn't hold the packet, we made a sling to secure it and put the chart on them. We tried to be as efficient as possible. I would put their arms around them, take a sheet and wrap it around them, put the chart in there, and make it soft and cozy next to their arms. What else could we do?" adds Rae Ann.

When her shift ends, she tries to sleep. At 1:00 A.M., she awakens to shouting. "Get Rae Ann. Her brother's here!" Rae Ann has two sisters and three brothers. Banking his boat next to the hospital's second floor is Walter Boasso, her brother and a Louisiana state senator. He has organized several volunteers to go to St. Bernard Parish to determine the conditions. The posse starts near the Claiborne area. It makes its way through the Ninth Ward, an area that extends 1 mile from its western Industrial Canal boundary to its eastern perimeter on the St. Bernard Parish border, and 1.5 miles from the Mississippi River to the northern border at Florida Avenue. In the Ninth Ward, people are screaming for help. The search mission becomes a rescue mission.

"He was hell-bent and determined to get to the hospital to see that we were OK, because he couldn't reach anybody by phone," says Rae Ann. "The last thing my sister-in-law heard was, 'The water's coming up,' and that was it. They never heard anything more."

Only one of the 20 boats reaches the hospital. Rae Ann races across the building. She shouts, "Lights, lights." People turn on their flashlights so she can avoid stepping on anyone. When she reaches the other side, a physician is talking with Walter.

"I took the doctor, pulled him over and I dove out the window. I grabbed my brother. I just started sobbing. It was, 'OK, somebody from the outside knows that we're alive! Somebody knows we're alive!' And I asked him, 'Walter, when are we going home?' He said, 'Tomorrow, baby. Tomorrow.' After seeing him kind of tear up, he said, 'We're going to get you out. We'll get you out tomorrow.' Then he asked the doctor, 'What do you need?'" As her brother promised, on Wednesday, the helicopters come. The 400 refugees who swam, came by boat, or whatever means they had to reach the hospital leave. The remaining patients are evacuated to the jail for care. Rae Ann says she felt she could breathe again, adding, "It was so stressful having patients because as a nurse you've got to take care of them. You couldn't focus on yourself or your needs. They needed you and they were your responsibility."

And then Rae Ann, her colleagues, physicians, and family members wait their turn. But it never comes. "We sit. We wait, but no one comes," she says. Where were they? Daryl helps dry out generators, get them running, and he hooks them up to electrical boards. Employees recharge their cell phones. It is about one or two in the morning on Thursday when Daryl finally reaches Walter on the phone.

Recounts Rae Ann, "He asks him, 'When are you coming to get us?' Walter says, 'What the hell are you doing there? What do you mean you are still there? They told me everybody was gone! Where are you?'"

Daryl replies that they are sitting on the hospital roof. The patients are gone. Walter asks if, on Thursday, Daryl and the others can get to the St. Bernard Port in Chalmette, located on the Mississippi River levee. Just as it had not flooded in 1965 for Hurricane Betsy, the port is dry. It is 2.65 miles from the hospital, typically less than 10 minutes away by car. But roads are underwater and submerged cars are water hazards. When daylight comes Thursday morning, there are over 20 people ready to leave with Rae Ann and Daryl. Among them is Rae Ann's colleague Lisa, who cannot reach her husband, an ER nurse at Methodist. Rae Ann convinces Lisa to go with her to the port. Once they reach Baton Rouge, Walter will help them find Lisa's husband. The group sets out in three boats. One will have to be towed.

"We all decided if we had to lie on top of each other, hold each other, strap ourselves down, we didn't care. We were getting out," says Rae Ann.

They take the canal located behind the hospital. They see a deer stranded on top of a partially submerged car. As they approach Jean Lafitte Street, they have to cautiously weave around trees, submerged cars, and other debris. Rae Ann sits at the front of the boat Daryl is steering. She guides him to avoid obstacles. In the distance, she sees another boat driven by someone in uniform. As it nears, Rae Ann sees that it is a police officer. They know the area is restricted for any traffic. Determined that they not be stopped, Rae Ann tells him she is the sister of Walter Boasso, who is waiting at the port for them.

"I am not a person who uses my brother's political status," she explains. "If you found out I was Walter's sister it is because you knew me, or you asked a direct question. I am not going to offer that information. That is not me."

The officer offers to escort them. He ties his boat and boards the lead boat. Rae Ann is relieved because now they have armed protection. They have heard about reports of gunfire. Finally they stop, but they are in the wrong place. They are by the Kaiser smokestack. It is almost four in the afternoon. They change course and head toward St. Bernard Highway, where the water level seems lower. A few of them get out and walk, while others remain with the boat in case they need it again. They slowly pull the boats. One boat hits something and takes on water. They find another boat that is abandoned. Soon they can no longer pull the boats by walking along the ditch. Rae Ann steps down into the black water. A few yards later, the officer says they should be able to feel the level of the street. Rae Ann falls. "He was just a second too late," she smiles. "I took a nose dive in the water. I came up quickly, thinking, 'What is in the water?' I didn't want to stress out, but I said, 'That's OK, you have a strong immune system.' We finally find where we need to go."

There is one last obstacle: a train. They will have to scale it to reach the port. They are not in the best of shape. They all try. One woman says she cannot make the climb. Daryl tells her the only way out is up. He pushes her up the rungs on the side of a railcar. They have arrived at the Katrina Camp, where hundreds of residents have taken shelter inside a warehouse. Families sit on blankets, surrounded by what few belongings they were able to salvage from their flooded homes.

"Walter worked himself to exhaustion through all of this," his sister says. "I found out later he got the Canadian Mounties to come down. . . . He was trying to do what he could for the people down here. This is where he was born and raised, like we were. We knew everybody. The principal at Chalmette High, got through on her cell phone to my niece, who was a freshman there. She said to Carol Ann, 'Tell your uncle Walter we are stuck here at Chalmette High.' So he is also trying to get them out. He was inundated."

Plans to drive to Baton Rouge change because there are so many with them. They will now leave by ferry. Despite reports of shootings at the Algiers Ferry, this is the best route out of the parish. When they reach a deserted ferry landing upriver, there is a school bus waiting for them. The group that left several hours ago from the hospital is now headed across the Crescent City Connection. They stop for meals ready to eat, water, and ice. As the bus heads west to the state capital, Daryl asks the driver to go faster than 40 mph. He obliges. It is almost midnight when the bus reaches their destination. As they disembark, Daryl offers the driver a tip.

"The guy says, 'Look man, let me tell you. I didn't want to tell you before, but I am not a bus driver. I am a janitor' . . . which is why he was only doing 40 mph. We all fell out laughing. Someone else who had to stretch themselves because of Katrina."

Reunited with their children and other family members, Rae Ann finally falls into a deep sleep. The following morning, her sister-in-law asks Rae Ann if she wants to see the school where her two children will be enrolled. Rae Ann walks into the school wearing the only clothes she has left—a t-shirt and pajama lounge pants. She sees a friend in the school corridor. "I just lost it. She lost it. We were sobbing. My husband starts crying. Then a girl that he grew up with is there with her kids. We all just started losing it in the middle of the place. People in Baton Rouge didn't know what they were getting with our arrival," she says.

Sunday comes, and Rae Ann realizes she needs a job. She calls Baton Rouge General and asks if they are hiring. They ask if she is a nurse. She tells them she is a registered nurse, displaced by the storm. They ask her to come in that same day for an interview and orientation. The next Monday, she starts a 12-hour shift.

Two weeks after the storm, she returns to Chalmette. Everything is still covered in mud. The stench is overwhelming. She and Daryl drive to the hospital. She has to retrieve one item from her office. It is a binder that contains her notes on formulas, medications, and lab values. She calls the binder her "brain."

"I told my husband if I am going to work in a hospital, I need my brain," she explains. "I find it. I burst out crying because it was almost like, 'OK, I can go on now. I have my tools to work.' And my husband didn't understand, but this is what I used every day. When someone would ask me something, I would say, 'Go look in my brain. It's over there.' It was all written down. . . . I could function. When I went back to Baton Rouge, once again that control thing, 'Now I have my brain, I can work.' That was part of my equipment."

In Baton Rouge, her family and her siblings rent two houses. Seventeen family members move into one house. At her new job, Rae Ann encounters some of her former patients. Six weeks on the job, her sister calls about their father. He is having chest pains. When he is brought to the ER, he is having a heart attack. He is admitted to the hospital. A few days after he is discharged, he goes into congestive heart failure.

"I am at work. They bring him. I take off of work. My mother is beside herself at this point. I don't know what I was running on, but I think work was an area I could control because I knew what to do there. That was my world that I could function in. The hospital staff was getting brand-new pumps . . . I was like, 'I can work these pumps.' They were all freaking out. I said, 'Y'all don't worry about it, *I can do this* . . . I can take care of patients and run the pumps. I can work here and can function right here.' Maybe that's what saved me—that I was still able to do this. I had a goal."

The demands of family eventually take precedence over her work, and Rae Ann resigns. She loves her work but cannot manage the two responsibilities. She is exhausted. That evening, she becomes ill with a 103° temperature. Having a history of arrhythmias, she realizes her heart is in bigeminy. She reaches her cardiologist, who is in Florida. He wants her to go to the hospital. She replies that that is not an option. He adjusts her medications; 3 days later, she recovers.

"I told him, 'I can't go to the hospital.' I figured it would kill my mother. My parents had dealt with enough. I was supposed to be functioning, not breaking down here. Perhaps when I quit, my body just needed a rest. By the fourth day, I was fine," she says.

By December, her family wants to return to St. Bernard Parish. Rae Ann wants to stay in Baton Rouge. Her father, in the early stages of Alzheimer's, has not ventured outside of the house since coming to Baton Rouge. Her mother stays at home to care for him. Rae Ann's parents want to go home, even though it means they and all of their children will have to rebuild. All of them qualify for a Federal Emergency Management Agency (FEMA) trailer, but Rae Ann says the small trailer did not accommodate her family of five. They buy a double-wide trailer, which they place on the land in Meraux where they will build their new home. In summer 2006, her parents move into a new house. By April 2008, Rae Ann and her family are in their new home.

Since 2008, she has been a nurse at a St. Bernard Parish elementary school. She admits that she would love to return to bedside nursing, but now is not the time.

"Right now, I can't," she offers. "I say I used to be a nurse, and even though I am a school nurse, you have to realize I was a cardiac nurse dealing with life-and-death situations. I had done that for so long. Here

I am giving magic ice and Band-Aids. It took me a long time to realize I can still be useful doing this."

She feels that so many other nurses went through a lot worse than she did and is aware how the experience has affected her, adding, "I can't take on any more. I've had enough of my own. I just pray they find some type of solace in what they do and that they're granted some peace."

And anyone who did not experience Hurricane Katrina, Rae Ann says, needs to know about it. "They need to understand first of all that we're people, too, and that when you are put in charge of someone else's life, the stress that is on you as a person and what that meant when nobody came to help until it was so bad. And FEMA to me just got in the way of so many efforts.

"I lost my job of 20 years. I lost my friends of 20 years. My sister moved to Georgia. I lost part of my family. Somebody had said, 'I don't understand why this is a big issue. I had a fire and lost my trailer.' Yeah, your neighbors helped you. Where are my neighbors? My neighbors need as much help as I do. Where was my priest? God only knows. My church, my congregation, where I would go for help. Where are my friends who would support me? We are all in the same boat. We are all neck-deep in water. We can't help each other. What do we do when all of your resources are all gone! You lost your job, your house. Some people go, 'Oh, they're material things.' Pictures of my babies. There are things that were precious to you and you saved. My wedding dress that I hoped one day my daughter would wear. They're all gone. You can never get that back. You have no choice. You start all over again."

Donna Sciortino

The water was like a big wave coming in. It was almost like a wave pool and started rising. It covered the entire first floor where the generators were. They blew in a half hour.

Donna Sciortino, LPN, became a licensed practical nurse in 2000. It was her second career, after spending 23 years with the Bell South Phone Company, where she went through the closing of three offices and then a divestiture. Her first nursing job was at a nursing home in Houma, Louisiana, but she found the work frustrating.

"I am a very hard worker, always have been," she begins. "I think my father taught me that when he worked two jobs quite a few years of his life. I feel that these people pay their dues all their life, and then to be in a nursing home where there is not enough staff was frustrating."

Currently Donna is working as a hospice nurse since Hurricane Katrina. Her children are her pets: dachshunds Zowie, Maggie, Abbie, and Isabella; bird Polly; and turtle Fred. She has been with her partner, Brenda, for the past 6 years; they reside in Mandeville, Louisiana.

In 2003, the native of St. Bernard Parish began working at Chalmette Medical Center. For Hurricane Katrina, she reports to work at the hospital's medical/surgical floor on Sunday, August 28, around three in the afternoon. Other employees did not come to work, but she understands their decision to evacuate with their families. It is a choice she wishes she had made.

"But I was glad to be there and do what I could do," she says. "Monday was when my week began, but I went to work on Sunday because I was told if I wasn't there on Monday I wouldn't have a job."

Before she leaves her home in Old Metairie to make the 20-mile commute to work, Donna calls her siblings, who live in St. Bernard and Violet. The youngest sister, Darra, has left for Monroe. Another sister, Debbie, will not evacuate. Nor will her brother Paul. Her brother, in frail health, is on the waiting list for a liver transplant. The interferon therapy he has undergone has weakened his body. Donna knows that the storm will be bad, and St. Bernard is not the place to be. On Sunday evening, Debbie's son brings boxes of fried chicken to Donna's unit.

"Debbie has cooked all her life, and the store was cleaning out their freezers before the storm. We had mountains of fried chicken that night," says Donna. Donna recalls Sunday at the hospital brimming with activity, "moving people around, getting everything settled, taking care of the patients, helping each other out." On the medical/surgical floor, there are 30 patients. Most of them are elderly. Some have family members with them. The hospital has a hurricane evacuation plan, but for Donna communication seems to be lacking.

"That was the frustrating part," she says. "Maybe there was a game plan. I did not know what it was. A lot of people were very frustrated. They had a lot of angry nurses before the storm came."

Before the weekend, several patients are discharged. Patients in the recently opened ICU have been transferred to Methodist Hospital. "It was a beautiful ICU," says Donna. "I was so proud of Chalmette Medical because they really came a long way with that new unit."

Patients on Two South, located at the front of the hospital, are moved to the rear of the hospital. On the second floor, the front area is designated as sleeping quarters for the nursing staff. On Sunday evening, the hurricane now hours away, Donna is fearful.

"I knew that we had generators if we had a flood on the first floor of the building," she explains. "That was what I was thinking. I knew we were going to have some water. I just could not imagine us not having any water from a storm that was so horrific. We had TVs and watched the reports until maybe two in the morning; everybody got rest. My shift started at seven that morning." The storm passes, and Donna recalls beautiful weather outside. The skies are clear. She considers ending her shift and going home. She wants to check on her house. Her plan is to pull medications needed for her patients and give the report to the next nursing shift.

"I was going to get fired if I didn't come in. I am here. I am going home. It is just after 8:30 A.M. and I go to pull my meds out of Pyxis. Then there comes the water," she recounts. "Oh, my God! I am on the second floor."

The water is coming from two directions. When the staff learns later about the citywide flooding, Donna assumes one source of the flooding for Chalmette is from a break at the Industrial Canal and the other is from the Mississippi River Gulf Outlet (MRGO). The MRGO is a 76-mile-deep draft navigation shipping channel that connects to the Gulf of Mexico.

"It looked like the waters were meeting each other at some point. I started screaming. I got a little hysterical. Everybody was waiting in line to pull their meds. Nobody was looking out the window. I said, 'Look out the windows!' The water was like a big wave coming in. It was almost like a wave pool and started rising. It covered the entire first floor where the generators were. They blew in a half hour. They still had people downstairs in the cafeteria and pharmacy. So, at that time, they start running up with everything from downstairs."

Employees scramble and move boxes of IV fluids, medications, and antibiotics from the pharmacy, which is relocated to the second-floor Pyxis room on Two North. Within an hour, the downstairs medical records area, lab, radiology department, and cafeteria are underwater.

It all seems surreal to Donna. Some people are hysterical. "I was so nervous when I saw the water come. What are we going to do? It was a matter of, 'Will the water go down, and when? What are we going to do with these patients?' No pumps. And then there was the heat."

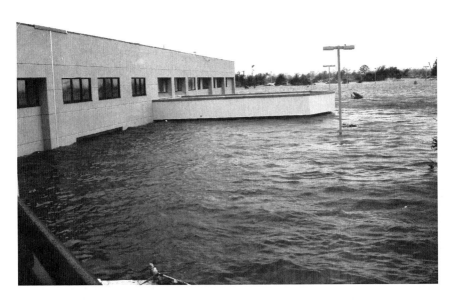

Flood waters cover the first floor of Chalmette Medical Center where over 400 people sought refuge after Hurricane Katrina. Photo by Bong Q. Mui, M.D.

Donna is able to make one phone call from the hospital roof. On her cell phone, she tells her partner that she is on the roof and the water is rising. Then the cell phone connection is lost. Bits of news trickle to the hospital staff. Someone hears that the levee behind the Lexington subdivision has collapsed. Twenty feet of water have engulfed the homes. By Tuesday morning, they hear what has happened to the city. Donna is resigned that they will have to wait their turn with the other hospitals before they are evacuated.

"I was hoping that at some point, it would start to recede, but where was it going to go? We really didn't know what was going on. We knew there was a levee break nearby and, of course, MRGO, so we got a double whammy."

By one o'clock that afternoon, the heat is becoming stifling. The second floor of the hospital belies the reality that the hospital is an island. Donna and others are concerned about the patients, especially the elderly, who are more susceptible to the heat.

"Of course, they were just miserable. It was horrific in there. I bet it was 110°. We started knocking out the windows. For some, they had to use a fire extinguisher to break the glass. Then the boats started arriving; we were getting people from Village Square—which had turned pretty much into a drug haven. It was quite frightening at that point. But we had to let them in because they were bringing these people for us to take care of them."

On Monday and Tuesday, Donna works and has little rest. If she sleeps more than 30 minutes, it is a luxury. On Tuesday morning, the hospital receives more residents, who have been rescued from the roofs of their flooded homes. Bedsheets are tied together and used to pull them from boats to the second floor. The hallways are lined with people. Room is made for the influx on Two North, located in the middle of the hospital. Donna says it was the least ideal place to be because there was no breeze there to give relief from the heat.

"We are wondering now what the plan is," says Donna. "I was quite unnerved. People were crying; some were hysterical. You are trying to take care of your patients, doing what you can do for them. You are giving antibiotics, running them by gravity, of course, because no pumps would work by then. Half of our patients needed to be hydrated. We had backed-up toilets, no organization about how to dispose of the human waste. People were using the bathroom on the floor in the patient's room. It was pretty nasty. It was a mess."

She says the physicians who were at the hospital worked tirelessly and recalls one, a recent addition to the medical staff, who helped keep everybody levelheaded. On Wednesday morning, the floodwaters start to recede slowly, revealing the tops of submerged cars.

There is also news about dry land at Paris Road and St. Bernard Highway. The plan is to bring the patients to the jail. They start moving them late afternoon. Each patient is wrapped in a bedsheet. Two people hold one end of the sheet, while two others hold the other end. Slowly, they inch their way down a ladder that is anchored on the boat floor and leaning against the wall below a second-floor window. The boat rocks in the water.

Donna says the entire transfer of patients to waiting boats below "was amazing. I was fearful we were going to drop a patient in the water and drown someone. I knew I was going to be OK, because I could swim."

She climbs down the ladder and boards a boat with two patients from the medical/surgical unit. She sits next to them, while supplies are loaded around them. Minutes later, the boat owner—a Good Samaritan who was one of many helping to rescue people—puts distance between his vessel and the hospital. It is almost 4:00 P.M. Donna sees fires coming from the Village Square site. She counts her blessings; there was no fire at the hospital, where it seemed everyone wanted to light up a cigarette.

At the corner of Judge Perez Drive, Donna has to get out of the boat to help pull it through water that reaches her knees. When they reach dry land, there are trucks waiting to bring them to the jail.

At the jail, the medical/surgical patients are hoisted onto the bunk beds in the jail cells. The task of hanging IVs and starting them is a challenge. IV bags are taped to the cinder block walls. Changing linens for patients in the top bunks is not easy. The cells seem to bake from the summer heat. There is no running water to wash their hands, and the supply of gloves is dwindling. In addition to her own patients, Donna and the other nurses tend to other patients and evacuees, who occupied any open space on the jail floor.

"You are taking care of others because you could smell the stool and the urine and you can only leave somebody in that for so long," she says. "But I have a joyful moment out of all of this. A lady who worked in the hospital respiratory department knew someone who was working at the Bell South building, two blocks from the jail. The building was air-conditioned by a generator, and we could rest there." But eventually, Donna begins to feel the effects of dehydration and heat. On Thursday, she feels faint. A colleague starts her on an IV of fluids. "I was about to pass out. It was so hot," she shares.

On Thursday, patients are evacuated via helicopter. The next day, September 2, Donna and the others also leave the jail. A convoy of pickup trucks takes them to the Violet Canal, where a shrimp boat is waiting for what Donna describes as an incredible route. She sees a dead cow near the side of the road. They need to reach the foot of the Paris Road Bridge. However, the main access road is underwater, so to reach their destination, the shrimp boat follows the Violet Canal to the bridge. People are shoulder to shoulder in the boat. With little protection from the sun, Donna says, they are, "cooked with sunburn."

At the foot of the bridge, they board a school bus, which makes its way along Chef Menteur Highway toward New Orleans. Some places along the road are covered with water, which reaches near the top of the bus tires. Donna contemplates what they would do if they are marooned on the road. Along the route, she sees fires, fueled by ruptured gas lines.

Donna tries her cell phone. She has no luck getting a signal. When the bus nears the Superdome, Donna crouches low in her seat because the passengers have been told there was shooting nearby. The bus continues heading west toward Gonzalez, Louisiana. It passes a convoy of military vehicles headed toward flooded New Orleans. Every few miles, Donna sees someone walking along the interstate. "I actually thought I saw a body, but I think I was hallucinating at that point," she says.

Finally, the bus arrives at Tanger Outlet Mall in Gonzalez. The mall parking lot is spotted with several yellow buses and hundreds of other people. Donna and her colleagues are given the option to continue on to Baton Rouge, where there is shelter at Jimmy Swaggart Ministries. Fatigued and weary, they decide to stay in Gonzalez.

"Fortunately, one of the nurses that we worked with had to be airlifted out, and they took her to the triage site by Lakeside. She was severely dehydrated, vomiting, low blood pressure. She was in touch with one of the nurses and said to come to her mother's home in Baton Rouge. I had my first bath in 6 days. It was wonderful."

From there, Donna reaches her partner and a friend, who had evacuated to Monroe. They drive to Gonzalez. When they see her, they ask if she is OK. She replies that she is not OK. During the 5-hour drive to Monroe, Donna lies down on the backseat and falls asleep. She feels safe but wonders about the rest of her family. Where are her sisters and brother? Her exposure to the bacteria from walking in the water has resulted in a severe case of cellulitis on her legs. One leg is swollen. At a Monroe hospital, she is treated and given a course of antibiotics.

In Monroe, she reunites with her sister Darra. They find their sister Debbie, who was airlifted to Houston, where she is among evacuees at the Houston Convention Center. They cannot find their brother. Two and a half weeks later, Donna gets a phone call from Zachary.

"He called me. I almost had a heart attack because I thought he was dead," she recounts. "I thought he had died and they just didn't find his body."

She learns later that her brother awoke to a flooded house when he put his hand in water that was inches from covering his bed. He tried to save his three pets, which were in the garage—a bird, a dog, and a gerbil—but could not. Alone in the house, he climbed the wrought iron lattice on the side of the house to reach the roof.

"When he got to the roof, he held on to the roof vent. He thought he was in a tornado. He said it was a black hole in the sky. My brother was very weak from the interferon. He swam to a two-story house in the next block, where someone picked him up in a boat and brought him to a store. On a Web site, there was a picture of a roof with his name and the names of five other men and the message they are alive. I have a copy of that on a canvas."

When Donna returns to her Metairie home, it is flooded with 3.5 feet of water, "just enough to make it a mess," she says. She moves across the lake to St. Tammany Parish, and in the second week of October 2005, she accepts a job at an area hospice. "So more death, more sadness," she says, but adds that returning to work helped her through the months following her ordeal. "I cried a lot. It took a while to process what I went through."

In August 2006, a year after Hurricane Katrina, her brother dies. It is the day after his 50th birthday. That same day, the family receives word that he has been approved for a liver transplant. Donna shakes her head. "After Katrina, it was months before my brother could find his transplant surgeon, who had relocated to Baton Rouge." She leaves the hospice job to take care of a friend's terminally ill husband. In 2008, she returns to work for hospice. Her sister Debbie rebuilds in St. Bernard. Donna hopes that for another major storm, Debbie will evacuate.

Donna says that part of her wants to leave it alone—Hurricane Katrina—and move on, "but you can be sitting somewhere and someone is going to say Katrina. I would like to hear about other nurses' stories. People probably won't believe half of what they're reading because it's so incredible. It is something you could not imagine happening. . . . If I had known that from the beginning. . . . The levees still are not fixed. They probably are never going to be. And that is frustrating."

Margie Palmeri

To listen to the messages and hear the panic in my children's voices, "Mom, please call us. We don't know where you are." That was difficult. I kept those messages on my cell for a very long time.

Margie Palmeri, RN, graduated from Louisiana State University (LSU) with a bachelor of science degree in nursing in 1981. She has been married for 26 years to Mark Palmeri; they have three children. She has been working in the medical field, in a hospital setting, since 1976, when she started working as a certified nursing assistant while a senior in high school. She worked for Chalmette General from 1981 to 1984, and for Humana Hospital from 1984 to 1990; she then returned to Chalmette Medical Center in 1990, and was there until Katrina (August 2005), when she lost "my home, my hospital, and my friends, rare and dear relationships I will never get back." She is currently working in a hospital in the greater New Orleans area.

Prior to Hurricane Katrina, Margie was the nurse manager of one of the hospital's medical/surgical units. She says that if a major storm directly threatened the area, their plan was to evacuate north of Interstate 12.

"We would go to a hospital in Lake Charles, Louisiana. We had done so with the critical patients before, for Hurricane Georges, transferring them by ground or air. The ambulance service the hospital used did not stop transporting until the very last minute, when it was no longer safe to be on the road." But Hurricane Katrina would be different. Because of its changing path, the Lake Charles hospital staff didn't know if they would have to evacuate patients should the storm steer westward. The plan at Chalmette Medical was to transfer patients and staff to Methodist, its sister hospital, which had more stories.

On Saturday, August 27, there is a brief meeting at the hospital for all departments. Everybody is on alert, ready to return if the storm changes its course. On Sunday morning, they return. Margie calls her staff to see who could report to work. When her three children were younger, she would bring them with her to the hospital for storms. But they were older—she had an eighth grader, a senior in high school, and one in college. They evacuate to Baton Rouge. Her husband reports to work at the New Orleans Marriott on Convention Center Boulevard, near the Mississippi River.

"At the hospital, the plan was that we were all going to evacuate to Methodist. Critical care was going to go first. Then we would take the patients who could go on a bus. After that, we would work on the rest. Well, this other ambulance service told us very early in the day they are not transporting patients. All of the ICU patients and staff were transferred to Methodist. Maybe a total of 60 patients, including those from ICU, got there."

The skilled nursing unit moves to Lakeland Hospital, on Bullard Avenue. Although there are no ambulances to continue the transfers, they continue bringing patients to Chalmette Medical Center's ER. Margie takes the news in stride: "I have been a manager for quite some time, and what we do is we hunker down, stay with what we have, and do what we have to do."

As patients arrive at the ER, they are held there on the first floor if they cannot be discharged. The others are quickly treated and released to their families so they can evacuate. The morning of Monday, August 29, there are reports of minimal storm damage to the hospital. The plan is to bring the patients in the ER to the second floor, starting at 7:00 A.M. But they begin moving them at 5:00.

"I remember my boss is on the phone with her brother, who called to ask her if she sees water. He heard the levees broke. She says, 'There is no water,' then turns and says, 'Oh, my God—here it comes!'"

As the streets flood, the staff scramble to get the last of the patients to the second floor. The employees calculate how quickly the water is rising. If the water threatens to reach the second floor, they will move everyone to the roof. If there is a full evacuation, it will not be the first time. In 1985, Chalmette Medical had a complete hospital evacuation to the then Humana Hospital in New Orleans East. At the time, Margie was pregnant with her daughter and on bed rest at Humana Hospital.

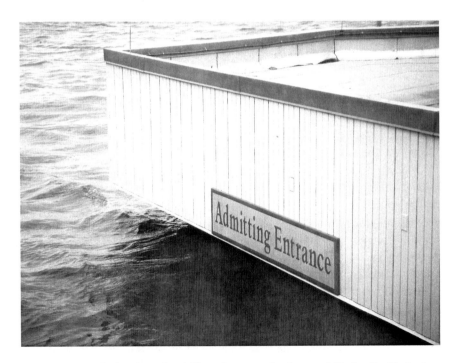

Flood waters are inches from the ceiling of a covered entrance of Chalmette Medical Center in St. Bernard Parish. Photo by Daryl Deroché.

Twenty years later, a second evacuation seems likely. The hospital dietitian sets up a temporary office with supplies on the second floor and begins meal planning. An area is designated for meal distribution. The water stops rising. Heat becomes another threat. But Margie says that everyone seemed to be grateful that they were there, "that they weren't sent off someplace else."

People are moved to the hospital's new wing located above the ER, which has a slightly higher elevation. The area has an exterior balcony. The staff breaks windows in the older part of the hospital to help air circulation. But the windows in the newly renovated wing do not break under the force of hammer and oxygen tanks. IV fluids are given to dehydrated patients and staff.

Midday on Monday, boats arrive, bringing rescued residents. Among them are children and infants. Having no nursery supplies, the staff improvise and use adult diapers for the infants. There are a few people in need of dialysis, but the hospital cannot provide the service. The plan is to evacuate them in the first patient exodus.

Margie describes the influx of people as "massive. We tried to keep those people away from the patient area. They were trying to go into patient rooms. The bathrooms were not working. We had what we called the shell area because it was another extension of the hospital that was not yet completed. It was a storage area with cement floors. That's where we housed those people."

There is no word when rescuers will come. On Monday, at midnight, a boat pulls up to the hospital, below the second-floor balcony. It is someone from the St. Bernard Sheriff's Department. They are looking for one of the hospital's physicians. "We looked at them and said, 'You can't take our doc. We need him here,'" says Margie. "But they were just checking on us and came to let us know they were setting up a MASH unit at the jail and wanted to make plans for the patients we had. The next morning, at 5:00 A.M., they are going to start getting the patients. So we first send the ER patients with the ER nurses and documents with each patient. About six patients went by boat late Tuesday night. We get a radio to communicate with the fire and police. The next day at 5:00 A.M., there is no one. Nobody, nothing."

When the sun comes up, the heat is unbearable. On Wednesday, August 31, over 200 evacuees who took shelter at the hospital leave by boat for the port. Now there are about 100 patients and family members in the hospital. The staff hear from the nurses who are at the MASH unit. There the conditions are much better and the land is dry. Around

10:00 A.M., patient evacuation starts. The first group to leave are the most critical patients, accompanied by staff that do not have families with them. A respiratory patient who cannot go by boat is airlifted from the hospital roof.

As patients leave, the employees form a human relay. They bring the patients from their rooms on stretchers to a room in the older wing, pass them through a broken-out window to the gravel roof, and wheel or carry them to the edge. From there, they are placed in bedsheets and lowered to the waiting boats. By Wednesday evening, the patients are all gone. And now over 100 family members of patients and employees remain. That evening, it is unclear how the rest will leave. Margie says the older nurses who had been through other storms seem to be OK. For others, the fourth day is wearing on them.

"Did I think we were not going to be rescued? No," replies Margie. "But we didn't know if we could go another week. People would come and say, 'We are coming back,' or they would send a helicopter, and they never came. And I had no word about my husband at the Marriott. We kept hearing rumors about people being shot, looting. He had a few policemen staying in the hotel with him, but I did not know if he was safe."

Daylight is waning, and Margie knows it will be another dark night. "You could still hear people on the roofs yelling, 'Help me, save me!' That was the hardest part, knowing people were out there. The night was pitch black," she says.

On Thursday, the last of the employees evacuate. Employees with children leave first. Margie and her colleague Bernie (Bernadette Is-bell) are determined that they will not evacuate by helicopter. "When the Chinook came, we did not know where they were going. Our chief executive officer and chief operating officer were the last to leave on it. They did not want to leave us, but we told them to take off; we are going in the boats to the port. We knew once we got everybody out that we could get to the port and from there make arrangements to get to Baton Rouge, where our families were. We were among the last ones out. It was near four in the afternoon when we left the hospital. When we left, I felt numb. I took pictures with my cell phone because I knew my family would want to know what happened. At night, while we were still at the hospital, we talked plenty about having no hospital. We talked about what we would do."

As their group of boats make their way to the port, one of the boats sinks. They find another boat and continue. In sections that are too shallow to allow the motors to run safely, a few of them step into waist-deep water and pull the boats. They come to their last roadblock—a train. They have to scale it to reach the port on the other side.

"I did not think I could do it, but we climb up and down the metal bars on the side of the train. And then we walk arm in arm to the port. We walked until we were finally out of the water. We were exhausted," Margie says. At the port, Margie can now retrieve the numerous text and voicemail messages that had been sent by her family since Monday. "To listen to the messages and hear the panic in my children's voices, 'Mom, please call us. We don't know where you are.' That was difficult. I kept those messages on my cell for a very long time."

From the port, they take a ferry west to Algiers, avoiding a more direct route because there are reports of shootings. At Algiers, they board a school bus. As it leaves the West Bank, they can see the Oakwood Mall burning. Later that evening, they arrive at Baton Rouge. Margie's husband is there. That morning, he had left the Marriott, escorted in a police caravan that protected them from the looters who were vandalizing downtown businesses. He tells his wife that as he left the hotel, he could hear the vandals breaking in.

Several days later, she learns that her brother is safe. When the storm surge flooded the area, he, his fiancée, and her mother swam to safety at a neighbor's home. He helped stranded residents but did not know of his sister's plight. He said that if he had, he would have checked on her.

For several months after the storm, Margie's husband commutes from Baton Rouge to New Orleans for work. The family returns to New Orleans and stays with a friend for 6 months, until they are able to move into their home in Marrero. Margie returns to bedside nursing because, she says, "It is all I knew." She believes she could have recouped from the loss of her home, which was completely flooded, if she had not also lost her community. "Everybody had losses in the parish, but it was not the same when Hurricane Betsy hit.

"Betsy flooded only part of the parish. We stayed with other family members while our house was rebuilt. We had that. Now, with Katrina, everything was gone. When you lost your job, you also lost all of your relationships with your job. I don't know how close other people were, but at Chalmette, we were family."

Today, she lives in Marrero and works at a New Orleans–area hospital on the West Bank of the city. And it is different. "It is not the physical, it is the emotional loss," she explains. "I drive back to the parish and I don't feel like I belong there. On the street where we lived, there are three houses on one side and four on the other, just in my block. Sometimes I miss it, but I feel like I don't belong. You don't belong here, you don't belong over there. When you get to be our age, your kids are grown. All the relationships that you had when they were growing up are scattered. At work, if someone was sick, you could call and somebody would take your place. Now it is different."

Today, Margie has been reunited with part of her Chalmette family; five of her colleagues from the medical/surgical unit at Chalmette Medical Center are working side by side with her.

Lisa Soileau

We were so lucky at Chalmette Medical that we had such a family environment because although it was a hardship, we were in it together. Nobody was out for themselves. Everybody worked together.

Lisa Soileau, RN, BSN, has been a nurse since 1985, when she graduated from the University of Southwestern Louisiana with a BSN. She initially worked at Southern Baptist Hospital for a short while, until she married and moved to North Carolina, where her husband was then working. When his job ended, they moved back to Louisiana, and Lisa accepted a position at Chalmette Medical Center. "It was a very small hospital, and yes, everyone knew everyone else's business, but we basically loved each other." It was her home away from home, the place from which she planned to retire. And then came Katrina. Life as they knew it was no longer. But move on they did, although the going has been very bumpy. She is currently working in a hospital in the greater New Orleans area. Her husband of 24 years is also a nurse. They have two children, Cory and Amber, who keep them on their toes.

On Saturday, August 27, 2005, Lisa Soileau and her family celebrate her birthday a day early. On Sunday morning, her husband, Philip, kisses her good-bye and heads to work at Chalmette Medical Center, where both of them are nurses. He is on staff at the skilled nursing unit, which is relocating to nearby Lakeland Hospital before Hurricane Katrina arrives.

Chalmette Medical Center was more than just the place where Lisa worked. It was her "other family" for almost 20 years of her nursing career. She believes she always wanted to be in nursing but first pursued a major in marine biology when she enrolled at the University of Southwestern Louisiana. She changed her major to physical therapy and, eventually, to nursing.

A seasoned veteran of storms, Lisa expects nothing extraordinary with Hurricane Katrina. As she finishes securing her home in an area she calls Old Chalmette, her mother arrives to collect Lisa's 13-year-old son, and 11-year-old daughter. Lisa reminds them to pack a 3-day supply of clothing and not to forget their schoolbooks. Her mother is taking them and their two dogs to an uncle's home in Baton Rouge. Eventually, they will end up in Arkansas.

"My mother would never leave for any storm. I don't know why she decided to evacuate, but I am thankful that she did," says Lisa. "Our pets are part of the family and surely they would have died. She and my children could have come to the hospital with me. It was very family-oriented, and families were invited to come. We lived two blocks from the Mississippi River, off St. Bernard Highway near the port, which is typically very high ground. I lived in that house since I was 2. For Hurricane Betsy, we got about 18 inches of water."

At two that afternoon, Lisa is at work at Chalmette Medical Center. March 2006 would mark her 20th year at the hospital, where she is a charge nurse for the 52-bed medical/surgical unit. On Sunday evening, there are 53 patients and about 200 people, including staff and their families. The patients are housed on the second floor, in the new wing, which has storm windows. Families occupy the North and South wings. Pets can stay with their owners. Lisa is focused on the tasks at hand. The hospital has a family atmosphere. People know each other. Someone stops by each unit with an ice cream cart and hands out ice cream to the families.

By Monday, when she readies for her day shift, the storm has passed. But at 9:30 A.M., the water rolls in. "When I saw this . . . what went through my mind is a movie we had recently watched, *The Day After Tomorrow*. Standing at the window and watching the water come in is unreal. The water pushed the cars against each other. It came in waves. It was just unbelievable. We didn't know what to think. We had no idea what was going on. Then we wondered how high the water would come."

In the stairwells, the water settles at the last two steps before the second floor, where a mobile pharmacy and dietary service have already been set up. The hospital's generators are underwater. Electricity and phone lines are out. And then the boats begin arriving, bringing the young and the old from the community. By the end of the day, Lisa says, there are over 400 people in the hospital. This startling influx of people is a concern.

"We did not know who they were, if they had guns or were seeking drugs," explains Lisa. "We had children in the facility. We knew our patients and families were OK. We were prepared for what we had as far as food and water, but when we got the extra people we were not prepared for that, so we had to ration what people got. We developed a [controlled portion] meal system; one meal was a slice of turkey, a scoop of vanilla pudding, and five ounces of water. We had probably 500 people to feed. We could not not take care of them. We were a hospital, but we were not a shelter. People were rescued and brought to us instead of being taken to dry land along the river. We would see sheriff's officers every once and a while walking through the hospital. We did see the National Guard."

Physicians made their rounds and would note orders in the patients' charts. "It was so unbearably hot because none of the windows where the patients were housed were able to be opened. We had some fanning brigades and children who would go through and offer water, juice, and fan patients. My godfather was a patient there at the time, so we had family and friends who came and did what they could. We kept people calm by talking, reassuring, and visiting with them."

On Monday evening, a helicopter lands on the hospital roof. Later, Louisiana state senator Walter Boasso arrives by boat. He is there to check on the facility and also on his sister, who is a nurse.

For Lisa and others, the hospital rooftop becomes a place of "release," where staff bring mattresses to sleep because it is cooler than inside the hospital. It is also the best place to get a cell phone signal. On Tuesday evening, Lisa borrows a cell phone to text her mother, knowing she will not know how to answer a text. Her message read, "Went through flood. I am alive."

"At night, it was so still," she recalls. "We heard people crying out for help. That was very difficult, to hear those voices calling for help and not be able to do anything. It was very distressing."

News reports are sporadic. It is hard to sort fact from fiction. Lisa learns later that families of employees believed the hospital was completely evacuated by Tuesday. They search for their loved ones, but learn the media reports are inaccurate.

"My most down period was one evening—we hear that gang members on the far side of the Claiborne Street Bridge are waiting for the waters to recede so they could come into town. That was the first time

I feared for my life. Knowing that we had drugs here and they were going to come. That was the scariest part."

The nursing staff work in three shifts. Attire is shorts, or scrubs cut above the knees. "Everybody worked together," she says. "Probably the hardest part of the whole thing is that we did lose patients. It was less than five patients, but that doesn't make it any easier. The hardest part was stopping. You reached this point where you could only resuscitate so far without means of a ventilator, and you can only ambu-bag somebody for so long. What do you do with the bodies in the extreme heat? Because it was a new wing, they had one portion undeveloped, so that is where we placed them." When evacuation starts on Tuesday, the locals who sought refuge are taken by boat to a dry part of the parish, from which they can walk to a staging area on the Mississippi River by the Port of St. Bernard. Volunteers and spouses of employees use their boats to help ferry them. They also scout for supplies and have success finding bottles of water. At the hospital, the bottles are washed for decontamination before distribution.

On Thursday, September 1, Lisa waits to leave the hospital. A boat approaches the hospital—she knows it is her brother Steve. His National Guard unit is based at nearby Jackson Barracks. "He climbed up to the roof. He came to make sure I was OK," smiles Lisa. "He had just purchased a home in Arabi, close to the river. It had about 5 feet of water in it. So, for my mother, it was a very emotional time for her, not knowing if her children were safe. Everyone in my family lost their home."

Despite the damage to Chalmette Medical, Lisa hopes it will eventually reopen. She takes comfort knowing that everyone did their best in a difficult situation. "We did what we had to do," she says. "At no time do I believe we were abandoned by the company. Not one time. The CEO was the last person to get on the helicopter. To me, that showed loyalty. He represented that company. At no time were we left alone."

On Friday, Lisa reaches Baton Rouge. It has been 5 days since she last saw her husband. That morning, Phil calls her. When he was airlifted from Lakeland, he, along with his administrator and six colleagues, were brought to the Interstate 10 and Causeway staging area in Metairie. They walked 8 miles to Williams Boulevard, where another employee's family met them and took them to Larose, Louisiana.

"It was such a relief to hear from him. 'I can start crying,'" says Lisa. "Just recently he told me he is finally not dreaming about those days at Lakeland. Unlike where I was, he felt very unsafe. Before I evacuated, I kept asking our CEO if he had any information from Lakeland. He said they had no word on their status. My husband was told that five employees at Chalmette Medical had died. There were no employees that died. So that was going through his mind, not knowing if I was dead or alive, and me not knowing if he was dead or alive. I remember sitting in the administration offices crying because I just didn't know."

The two are reunited in Baton Rouge. They drive to New Iberia, Louisiana, where a stranger from Arkansas (where her family had evacuated) offers to fly down to New Iberia to pick them up in his fixed-wing plane and fly them back to Arkansas. For a year, Lisa's focus is on her children. Not wanting to uproot them, she remains in Arkansas. In February 2006, her husband returns to New Orleans. In June, at the close of the school year, she and the children return home. She is the last member of her family to move back. At their home in Chalmette, the waterline stopped 2 inches below the first-floor ceiling. They go through their savings to recover from their losses. They decide to leave the area and relocate to Pearl River, Louisiana.

In October 2006, Lisa accepts a position at a New Orleans–area hospital. For 2 decades, she had been a charge nurse, working as a physician liaison and processing orders. Her direct patient care was minimal. "That was my job, and I was good at it," she says. "But I didn't provide direct patient care other than supervising and assisting with general or difficult procedures. I am a creature of habit, and going into the unknown created much turmoil for me."

But Lisa made the transition to her new work as a unit-based educator. She works three 12-hour shifts. Working again with her Chalmette Medical Center colleagues has been a lifesaver. "We were so lucky at Chalmette to have such a family environment because, although it was a hardship, we were in it together. Nobody was out for themselves. Everybody worked together," she says.

And she is ready to work during another storm "because that is what I signed up to do. I would do it again tomorrow. That is just what we did."

Bernadette Isbell

We didn't just lose our houses or our possessions. We lost our community and our anchor.

Bernadette Isbell, RN, graduated from the University of Southwestern Louisiana in December 1993 and started working at Chalmette Medical

Center that same month. She has been married 13 years and has five children and one grandchild. Her mother worked at Chalmette Medical when it opened, and then retired. She has the same plans because "we all seemed like family." She worked as a case manager at the time of the storm—since then, she has chosen to go back to floor nursing and loves it. She does not exactly know "where my nursing career will take me" but is hopeful that one day, there will be a hospital in Chalmette for her to work at again.

"For me, we were more than coworkers. We were comrades before Katrina happened," she says. "It was a special place to work. We were always looking out for each other, no matter what happened. You stubbed your toe, someone was there for you. Everybody helped each other through illnesses and through joyous times of weddings, childbirths, watching your children grow. Whether it was a hurricane or whatever, we always treated each other that way."

So when she came to work the Sunday before Hurricane Katrina, she felt assured that her colleagues would be there to offer support. "Monday I talked to my husband at 7:10 in the morning. I told him I was good, getting ready to serve breakfast to the patients. I would probably be home late that evening or tomorrow because I was an ancillary person. When I finished serving breakfast, someone says the first floor is almost gone and the water is coming in.

"I am like, 'What?' It didn't register to me that I wouldn't have a job for a long time or the hospital would even close," she offers. As soon as the water starts rising, people from the neighborhood seem to pour into the hospital. They hoist themselves over the hospital balcony. Unsure when they could fully evacuate the hospital, the staff distribute numbered armbands to everyone. Bernie says they did not run out of food or water. They hear that the majority of St. Bernard Parish is flooded. Bernie is confident that her home in Violet is underwater. "I knew the house was gone, but what could you do?" she asks.

"Tuesday we had people like the National Guard coming to us and telling us they'll come back, but never show up. So everybody in the hospital had an armband and a number. When mealtime came, we checked the numbers off a list and told them, 'If you use someone else's number, you will not get a meal.'"

Not knowing when they would leave was not as challenging as the heat and ensuring comfort for the patients. "I can remember being in a room with a nurse, assisting her. She was in the middle of changing a dressing. After 20 minutes in the room, I stepped out for a minute because

I just had to take a breath. She continued with the dressing change—
I tell this to emphasize how these nurses cared for these patients dear
to me."

Administration keeps the staff informed on a regular basis. There
are meetings throughout the day. The National Guard stops by in the
afternoon late Monday. On Tuesday morning, Bernie expects to see her
husband, but he does not show. She becomes concerned. He had stayed
at their home located 2 miles from the hospital. A sheriff's boat comes
by to check on the hospital. A helicopter lands on the roof Tuesday. The
hospital chief operating officer leaves on it but returns the next day.

Around 2:00 P.M. on Tuesday, Bernie's husband arrives at the hospital. He had spent Monday night at the shelter set up at Chalmette High
School. He says the situation there was horrendous and vows to sleep in
the woods, if necessary, but he will not go back there. The next day, he
helps ferry patients to the MASH unit set up at the parish jail.

Late Wednesday night, she receives a text message from her son. It
reads, "Where are you?" Standing on the hospital roof, she tries to get a
signal on her cell phone. "For some of the cells we could use the boat to
recharge the batteries," she says. "I text him back, 'OK, stay where you
are.'" When employee evacuation begins, there is a buddy system.

"As we put people on the helicopters, we made sure they had a few
dollars in cash, because some people didn't come with anything or had
left it in their purse," explains Bernie. "So we pooled our cash and we
made sure they had a buddy with them. We told them, 'This is your
buddy; try to stay with this person, so wherever you go you will at least
have one other person with you.' We knew one was on medication. We
sent him with bottled water and crackers in case he was stuck somewhere for a period of time so he had something to eat and hydrate and
take with his medicines."

On Thursday, Bernie and her husband are among the last to leave
the hospital. They reach the Port of St. Bernard and, from there, go to
Algiers, and then to Baton Rouge. Late that night, they reach the state
capital. When he removes his wet shoes and socks, Bernie is shocked
by her husband's red and swollen feet. He has difficulty walking and is
diagnosed with a circulatory problem. He is treated with bed rest and
fluids.

Home for now is in Gretna, Louisiana, while they rebuild their
home in St. Bernard Parish. Starting over is a slow process, but Bernie
is philosophical.

"Anything can happen to any of us any given day. We have hurricanes, other people have earthquakes. We have some warning prior to our storms. Many of us talked about retiring maybe at age 70 because we enjoyed so much working together. Those relationships are precious. We didn't just lose our houses or our possessions. We lost our community and our anchor."

In October 2005, a month after the hurricane, Bernie started working as a case manager at a West Bank hospital. Her friend Margie Palmeri joined the staff that November.

"And then as soon as she came here, a few of the other nurses came. I used to do paperwork nursing, but I said, 'I will give that up and work on the floor to be with them.' I do three 12-hour shifts. It is a tremendous thing for me to come to work and see those faces."

The future of another Chalmette Medical Center remains uncertain. Should it reopen, Bernie says, there is a floor staff ready for work. "We have an entire unit staffed for 12-hour shifts. We have a director, a charge nurse, and floor nurses to take care of 36 patients."

7   Lessons Learned

This chapter describes the lessons learned from a national disaster such as Hurricane Katrina. Reports with assessments from Congress, state governments, and independent agencies are highlighted. An interview with Sandy Rosenthal, the founder and executive director of Levees .org, details the safety of the levee protection system, not only locally in the greater New Orleans area, but across the nation. Several reports and investigations will provide information about the failures that occurred because of Hurricane Katrina. These reports include *The Federal Response to Hurricane Katrina: Lessons Learned* (White House, 2006), *A Failure of Initiative: Final Report of the Select Bipartisan Committee to Investigate the Preparation for and Response to Hurricane Katrina* (H. Rep. No. 109-377), and *Hurricane Katrina: A Nation Still Unprepared* (S. Rep. No. 109-322).

The *Federal Response* report (White House, 2006) provides a perspective on Hurricane Katrina and 125 recommendations for improvement. The report cites 17 critical challenges that were identified after an investigation of the federal response to Hurricane Katrina. The purpose of this report was to identify the issues and gaps that had been problematic and determine how to improve disaster preparedness and response at federal, state, and local levels of government. Key improvements in these areas will require changes in policy, planning, and preparedness of the nation; use of military resources in an integrated manner; communications, logistics, and evacuations; search and rescue; safety and security of the public; health and medical support of the public; human services; care and housing for the masses; public communications; impact assessment and critical infrastructure; environmental hazards and removal of debris; foreign assistance; nongovernmental aid; training, exercises, and lessons learned; homeland security; professional development and education; and preparedness for citizens and the community (White House, 2006).

Each of these critical challenges describes lessons learned and recommendations for improvement. One example is communication, which was a critical challenge resulting from Hurricane Katrina. The communications infrastructure of the greater New Orleans area was decimated, leaving hundreds of thousands with communications challenges. The report calls for the development of a National Emergency Communications Strategy that supports the operability and interoperability of communications (White House, 2006). The state of Louisiana has been working diligently since the storm to implement strategies to improve the communication infrastructure. Such improvements include adoption of the National Incident Management System by hospitals, establishment of a regional structure to facilitate response, identification of a hospital emergency preparedness coordinator, implementation of the EMSystem, implementation of ongoing drills at the state and city levels, and identification of communication systems for redundancy (Louisiana Hospital Association, 2007).

Another critical challenge was obtaining needed supplies and equipment during and after Hurricane Katrina. The *Federal Response* indicates that federal resource managers had a difficult time determining what resources were needed, what was available, and where to obtain and send resources since situations in the facilities were constantly changing. The report recommends that a coordinated effort among state, local, public, and private sectors be developed through a comprehensive logistics plan for emergencies, and that the federal government be capable of conducting a large-scale logistics operation (White House, 2006). Locally, many hospitals have developed contracts with vendors to bring in needed supplies for a specific time period. The regional coordinator designate will support and coordinate the process of resource availability in each region throughout the state.

The *Federal Response* (White House, 2006) provides a synopsis of those areas that, after being investigated, fell short of achieving a high level of success. It is the intention of the report to address these critical challenges so that, in the future, the government will be better prepared to protect its citizens.

The U.S. House of Representatives approved H. Res. 437 on September 15, 2005, which created a select bipartisan committee to investigate the preparation and response to Hurricane Katrina. The result of the investigation was presented in a document released in 2006, titled *A Failure of Initiative: Final Report of the Select Bipartisan Committee to Investigate the Preparation for and Response to Hurricane Katrina* (H. Rep. No. 109-377, 2006; U.S. House of Representatives, 2006). A summary of the findings of the committee includes the conclusions that the levee protection was not built to shield the city from severe hurricanes; the failure to completely evacuate patients and citizens led to preventable deaths and suffering; the National Response Plan was not fully executed in a timely manner; the Department of Health Services, the Federal Emergency Management Agency (FEMA), and the state were not prepared for this event; there were major communications failures and no sufficient backup systems; and lack of coordination and control at all levels of the government and the ultimate collapse of law enforcement created a lack of safety and security.

The congressional report (S. Rep. No. 109-322, 2006) titled *Hurricane Katrina: A Nation Still Unprepared*, conducted by the Senate Committees on Homeland Security and Governmental Affairs, identifies four overarching factors that contributed to the many failures that occurred as a result of Hurricane Katrina. The factors include that the government did not adequately prepare for this type of catastrophic event; government officials made poor decisions on various issues during and after the hurricane; systems throughout the government failed; and there was poor leadership at all levels of government. The report addresses evacuation, military support, law enforcement, and health care. The report emphasizes the issues that Louisiana faced with the Louisiana Office of Homeland Security and Emergency Preparedness, and the Office of Emergency Preparedness for New Orleans in particular, on issues concerning the evacuation of citizens and patients and the levee system. The report provides seven recommendations, including replacing FEMA with an organization that is stronger and more capable than the National Prepardness and Response Authority.

THE NATION'S LEVEE PROTECTION SYSTEM

What's past is prologue.
—*The Tempest*, William Shakespeare

In the past century, New Orleans has been flooded six times: in 1915, 1940, 1947, 1965, and 2005. Following Hurricane Betsy in 1965, Congress authorized the Lake Pontchartrain and Vicinity Louisiana Hurricane Protection Project in the Flood Control Act of 1965. The project called for the construction of flood walls, levees, and control structures to provide hurricane protection around Lake Pontchartrain to the parishes of Orleans, Jefferson, St. Bernard, and St. Charles.

In its summary of the September 25, 2005, report, *Army Corps of Engineers: Lake Pontchartrain and Vicinity Hurricane Protection Project*, the U.S. Government Accountability Office (GAO) noted that since the project began, there have been project delays and increases in costs. These are attributed to changes in design due to technical issues, concerns about environmental impact, legal challenges, and local opposition to some parts of the project (U.S. Government Accountability Office, 2005; Infrastructure Security Partnership, 2002–2009). Forty years after its commencement, the project is not completed.

According to the American Society of Civil Engineers Hurricane Katrina External Review Panel's report, *The New Orleans Hurricane Protection System: What Went Wrong and Why*, there were breaches at 50 locations in the city's levee system (American Society of Civil Engineers [ASCE], 2007).

Around 5:00 A.M., there was a breach in the east bank of the Industrial Canal I-wall. A significant storm surge level at the Intercoastal Waterway was created by the strong east–west winds of the storm. By 6:30 A.M., levees on the south side of New Orleans East were overtopped and breached (ASCE, 2007). At about 6:30 A.M., a breach was observed in the I-wall, in Orleans Parish, of the 17th Street Canal (ASCE, 2007). At about 7:00 A.M., there was a breach in the London Avenue Canal I-wall near Mirabeau Avenue in Gentilly (ASCE, 2007). Almost an hour later, there was a second breach on the London Avenue Canal, near Robert E. Lee Boulevard (ASCE, 2007).

In St. Bernard Parish, flooding was contributed by storm surge overtopping the Forty Arpent Canal levee. By Thursday, September 1, over 80% of the metropolitan New Orleans area was flooded (ASCE, 2007).

Immediately following the hurricane, there were five investigations, three major and two minor: The Army Corps of Engineers sponsored the Interagency Performance Evaluations Task Force (IPET), and two independent studies were conducted by the University of California at Berkeley (Independent Levee Investigation Team) and Louisiana State

University. Two minor studies were conducted by FEMA and the insurance industry.

On November 2, 2005, the Homeland Security and Governmental Affairs Committee held its fifth hearing addressing why the levees in New Orleans failed. Expert witnesses included Ivor Van Heerden, PhD, Louisiana team leader, forensic data gathering; Paul Mlakar, PhD, PE, senior research scientist, U.S. Army Engineer Research and Development Center; Raymond B. Seed, PhD, team leader, National Science Foundation; and Peter Nicholson, PhD, team leader, Levee Assessment Team, American Society of Civil Engineers (Homeland Security and Governmental Affairs Senate Committee [HSGAC], 2005a).

On December 15, 2005, the committee held its ninth Katrina hearing. Focus was on the key government agencies responsible for the operation and maintenance of the New Orleans–area levees (HSGAC, 2005b).

In early June 2006, the Corps released IPET, a 6,000-page report on the failed levee system. At a news conference, Lieutenant General Carl Strock, commander and chief engineer of the Corps, acknowledged that design defects in the New Orleans–area levee system caused the majority of flooding during Hurricane Katrina.

One year later, Major General Don Riley, the Corps' director of civil works, contradicted Strock's acknowledgment and suggested that the levee breaches could not have been prevented by the Corps. A Corps-financed report titled *Hurricane Protection Decision Chronology* was released on July 11, 2007. The report traces the history of key decisions that led to the catastrophic levee failures after Hurricane Katrina (Wooley & Shabman, 2007).

The Independent Levee Investigation Team called the performance of the New Orleans regional flood protection system unacceptable and cited engineering issues related to its failure. It noted that no one group or organization was solely responsible for the August 29, 2005, levee failures, which had catastrophic results, and noted the need for interactive and independent expert technical oversight and review (Seed et al., 2006).

Sandy Rosenthal

Most major American cities lie partly in a floodplain. It is important to take this discussion outside of New Orleans because

43% of the American population lives in counties protected by levees.

Sandy Rosenthal, then 49, founded Levees.org, a flood protection nonprofit with a mission of education—that metro New Orleans was destroyed primarily by civil engineering failure, not a weather event. Levees.org is a grassroots group and accepts no funding from stakeholder industries. Levees.org has grown to over 23,700 supporters, with satellite locations in Florida, California, and Illinois. The Associated Press recently dubbed Levees.org "an influential citizens group." In late 2007, Ms. Rosenthal gave up her job as an advertising executive to devote herself full-time to the demands of being an activist leader. She graduated from Mount Holyoke College cum laude in 1979 and received a master's degree in business administration from Tulane University, New Orleans, in 1981. Ms. Rosenthal has been a New Orleans resident since 1980, has been married for 29 years, and has three adult children.

When Sandy Rosenthal evacuated her New Orleans home and headed to Lafayette, Louisiana, to get out of the way of Hurricane Katrina, she planned to be away for 3 weeks. A discussion with a resident from Alexandria would become the catalyst of what she would do when she returned home.

"I was trying to explain to this man that if the levees had held, we would have been fine," she recounts. "It was an engineering failure. He said, 'No, the levees are fine. They were built right. It was just that the storm was too big and New Orleans is below sea level and you shouldn't have been there in the first place.' And he was ugly about it. Here I am, living in Lafayette, evacuated from my house, and having this argument. Little did I know, he was the best person I could have talked to because if you go outside the state, it's not that bad. They may not be the most sympathetic, but they're not going to be ugly about it. They're not going to call us stupid for living here. They're not going to call us imbeciles for our wish to rebuild. So I should thank him. That was the best thing that could have happened."

On December 1, 2005, Sandy Rosenthal launches Levees.org, a nonprofit group that she oftentimes finds acting as a watchdog group over the Army Corps of Engineers because the group corrects misinformation loudly and publicly. The organization's mission is to educate American citizenry about what happened on August 29, 2005, and why.

Levees.org began with Sandy and her son as the organization's Web master. By spring 2009, its membership was 23,700, and growing. The response to Levees.org was a surprise to its founder.

"I had always thought big in order to educate America," she explains. "You can't get big if you don't think big. But I didn't know it would shake out the way it did. I didn't know I would be taking on the United States Army Corps of Engineers. I didn't know I would be taking on the very powerful American Society of Civil Engineers and others. I didn't know I'd be taking on the media industry itself."

When she founded Levees.org, Rosenthal was unaware that metro New Orleans's levees are federally designed and built, and the local citizens are responsible only for taxation and for maintenance after they're constructed. "The 17th Street Canal levee was finished, but there are many levees still under construction," she explains. "I didn't find that out until I read the GAO report in mid-December 2005," she adds.

"By law, the levees are designed and built by the Corps in metro New Orleans. We can't just go and build our own levees. And that's what people don't realize. Since I founded Levees.org, I am finding that citizens can make a difference. What I did know is that the levee failures here were federally caused, and the only organization that can help us is the federal government—Congress. And there is no way the Congress will be sympathetic and send us the assistance we need if the American people think this is our fault. Because Congress does what the American people want. One hundred percent of the levees in the New Orleans area are federal."

On January 3, 2007, Levees.org announced its campaign for the 8/29 Investigation Act, an independent analysis at the local, state, and federal levels of the flood protection failures and organizational component during Hurricane Katrina. The executive director says that the 8/29 Investigation Act calls for an objective look and comprehensive analysis of flood protection projects and the effects of coastal erosion. It would also examine how federal water projects in the upper Midwest and High Plains may have caused Louisiana to lose land that is no longer a natural buffer against hurricanes.

On June 11, 2007, the Louisiana legislature unanimously passed a resolution calling for the 8/29 Investigation Act. In response to those critics who claim that New Orleans should not be rebuilt because it is vulnerable to flooding, Rosenthal notes that 39 of America's 50 largest cities live partly on floodplains.

"Most major American cities lie partly in a floodplain," she says. "It is important to take this discussion outside of New Orleans because 43% of the American population lives in counties protected by levees. That was announced June 15, 2008 [at the Congressional Hazards Caucus]."

On February 24, 2006, California governor Arnold Schwarzenegger declared a state of emergency for the state's levee system and signed an executive order for the state's Department of Water Resources to repair 24 erosion sites in Colusa, Sacramento, Solano, Yolo, and Yuba counties (Environmental News Service, 2006).

"Dallas has been informed by the Corps of Engineers that their levees are in terrible condition; they all need to be rebuilt and they are in great danger of flooding," Sandy offers. "The residents are saying, 'What?' In fact, we in New Orleans would have welcomed such advance warning. In Sacramento, right after Katrina, Governor Schwarzenegger called for a check of the state's levee system and found that they were in worse condition than what we had here. If a seismic event broke their levee, they would be in big trouble. So what happened? They voted for billions of state money to fix the federal levees. But they have the capital. They can do that, and Texas probably has the capital to do the same."

Rosenthal is passionate in her quest to have accountability from the Army Corps of Engineers. "To make them accountable is easy. The citizens have to demand it. When you go to Japan, the fish is really fresh. You order sashimi and the fish is still moving. Because the Japanese demand it and won't eat anything that is not absolutely fresh. In the States, our fish has been sitting around for days. Well, it's the same with our levee protection. You must demand it. I've been working on this for 3 years, and I do not hear enough citizen participation. I don't see enough citizen involvement."

She sees two major reasons for this lack of response. One is political. "People during the last administration saw Levees.org's efforts as antigovernment. I have been called antigovernment. The other reason is a feeling of hopelessness. 'What can I do as a citizen?' Talk about you can't fight City Hall! This is a thousand times harder than fighting City Hall. So I think it's a feeling of people believing it's useless and hopeless. But I am not giving up. And each day, we get more members and become stronger, and anything worth having is not built overnight. This is unprecedented. Nothing quite like this has ever happened."

On April 20, 2009, the Mississippi River Gulf Outlet (MRGO) trial started in federal court. Plaintiffs have charged that the Army Corps of Engineers's failure to properly build and maintain the MRGO eroded protective wetlands and caused massive flooding, which destroyed their homes and businesses (Finch, 2009). The Corps cites the levees as the cause of flooding in St. Bernard Parish and the Lower Ninth Ward.

A 1928 federal law gives the Army Corps of Engineers immunity from liability for damage caused by its flood protection projects. However, with this lawsuit, the Corps has no immunity under law involving a navigation project. The Corps has maintained that MRGO had minimal impact on flooding from Hurricane Katrina in 2005 (Finch, 2009).

The MRGO, constructed by the Corps, opened in 1963 as a shortcut for large ships traveling between the Gulf of Mexico and the Industrial Canal in New Orleans. The 76-mile-deep draft navigation channel is 40 miles shorter than traveling the Mississippi River between the Gulf of Mexico and New Orleans (Carter & Stern, 2006). It was officially deauthorized on June 5, 2008 (U.S. Army Corps of Engineers Team New Orleans, n.d.). Three days later, MRGO was officially closed to boats. A permanent barrier at Bayou La Loutre near Hopedale was completed by summer 2009. The rock structure base is 450 feet wide, tapering to 12 feet at the top. It is 950 feet long and 7 feet from the water's surface. The barrier is made of 430,000 tons of rock that covers 10 acres of the channel bottom.

"We need the 8/29 Investigation Act. It was refiled for 2009, but we still have a long way to go," explains Sandy. "There are several things that are going to happen. With the MRGO trial, a lot of information is going to come out that we didn't know before. The National Academy of Sciences has not yet finished their peer review of the Corps' self-study. They are going to be unhappy with what they find. The Corps' self-study will not hold water on either a technical or ethical basis. It will fall short of expectations. There is too much conflict of interest. That will be another reason for the 8/29 investigation."

The Levees.org founder and executive director says accountability and transparency will come with peer review. "We need outside agencies looking in," she says. "The Corps controls billions of dollars annually, and for years they had no peer review of significance. Last year, it was passed into law that they will have peer review, but it's only on how water projects are built, not how they are chosen."

She feels the reason that part did not pass "is because Congress would have to give up its power in choosing which projects are done. But the citizens can demand it, and if enough citizens demand it, then it gets done. It all gets back to the fresh fish. If you want fresh fish, you will get it. The guy with the old fish, no one will buy it."

The levee board consolidation, she adds, took away the board's assets—"their marina, all their land, their police. Now they have no assets. What the levee board should have are inspectors watching the levees' construction, making sure they're done right. We don't have the money to pay someone to do that."

She offers that while many people outside Louisiana feel terrible about the massive devastation from Katrina, "for some, in order to deal with that feeling, they welcomed evidence that our losses were somehow our fault because it makes them feel better. That way they can dismiss it and move on. It gives them the opportunity to heal from it. Also the media looked about for people who were willing at that time to feed the frenzy to blame New Orleans for the flooding. These media-seekers' information was wrong, but the media drank it up, printed it, and sent it out. Much of the American people wanted to hear it. So the media fed it. It was comforting to believe our woes were our fault."

After Katrina, Congress authorized construction of new lakefront pumping stations at the mouths of the 17th Street, Orleans Avenue, and London Avenue canals. Two options have been considered. The first one would replace the temporary pumping stations with permanent ones. During a hurricane, these pumps would be used and would have to work in tandem with much older Sewerage and Water Board pumps on the other ends of the canals. During normal rainfall, the new pumps would not be used (Grissett, 2009).

Option 2 calls for permanent lakefront pump stations and would deepen and pave the outflow canals so water would gravity-flow to the lakefront. The permanent lakefront pumps would become all-purpose, year-round stations. The Corps has acknowledged that Option 2 is the better plan, technically and operationally superior, but cites Option 1, adhering to a congressional mandate to provide the cheapest possible flood protection (Grissett, 2009).

"It is historic. The Corps of Engineers tends to lowball, to understate, and to underestimate the costs of projects they want to do, and they tend to astronomically inflate the projects they don't want to do," notes Rosenthal. "Cutting costs to build poor protection leads to higher costs to rebuild. At least America gets that now."

Louisiana's congressional delegation opposes the Corps' choice. U.S. Senator Mary Landrieu (D-Louisiana) recommends changing the current way the Army Corps of Engineers operates in developing water projects and considers having a new agency or combination of agencies to handle levee concerns (Schleifstein, 2009).

At the time of this writing, the Corps is moving forward with Option 1 for the pump stations, despite growing opposition that includes the Louisiana Coastal Protection and Restoration Authority and the Southeast

Louisiana Flood Protection Authority. The Corps says that Congress did not authorize appropriate money for such expanded projects (Grissett, 2009). Until the New Orleans–area flood protection is finished, Rosenthal says, she will hold her breath each hurricane season from June 1 to November 30—and so will the residents of the metropolitan New Orleans area.

Cynthia

As bad as the situations are at the hospitals, hospitals are still considered to be safe havens. You've got buildings with supplies, with educated people. I think the staff at some of the hospitals got very upset that the government didn't rush in to rescue them. But the fact of the matter is that part of evacuation has not changed. A hospital still has to be prepared to stand in place 5–7 days because they remain a safe haven. The first tier of rescue will be for the people on tops of rooftops and buildings.

Cynthia, who is an RN, is the administrative designated regional coordinator for hospital emergency preparedness and response in Louisiana Region 1, the greater New Orleans area. As a registered nurse, she has over 20 years of experience, from staff nurse to chief nursing officer/chief operating officer. Additionally, she spent 12 years in the Army Nurse Corps and U.S. Army Reserve, as a member of a combat support hospital. Cynthia was a practicing trial attorney and, for 12 years, was a senior attorney at the Medical Center of Louisiana at New Orleans, in charge of contract administration. She has served as president of the Plaquemines Parish Bar Association and is a member of the Louisiana State Bar Association's Legal Malpractice Insurance Committee. After Hurricane Katrina, Cynthia was an original member of the Greater New Orleans Healthcare Taskforce, which was created to assist in restoring health care services in Region 1. She was the cochair of the Bring New Orleans Back Health and Specialty Care Subcommittee and a member of the Healthcare Redesign Collaborative. She serves as a representative on the Louisiana Emergency Response Network.

On Friday, August 26, at 9:00 A.M., Cynthia holds a meeting at the Metropolitan Hospital Council of New Orleans with representatives from Region I hospitals. She reviews with hospital representatives their emergency preparedness plans. She is concerned that Hurricane Katrina may come their way.

"There was a lot of bravado and the mind-set that the storm would not hit Louisiana," Cynthia recounts. "This gave me great concern. The last time we had a serious threat was Hurricane Georges. That was their reference. Georges was coming toward us but then turned to Biloxi, Mississippi. I was saying, 'Wait a minute—you have to go back to your hospital and make sure you are prepared, because this thing could turn to us.' The response was, 'We'll be fine.' So I made several calls because I was on pins and needles. I am not feeling as comfortable as they were."

Throughout the day, she calls the emergency preparedness coordinator at the Veterans Administration Hospital (VA) in downtown New Orleans. He is the volunteer DRC in Region I. Cynthia knows his information source is direct from federal officials. Despite his reassurances, Cynthia tells him she is not feeling good about the situation.

"What was really concerning me was again this notion about being prepared at the hospitals, but they were really not thinking of having to be prepared. They had not done the normal things that we do in advance of a storm, such as canceling clinics. Friday, they were having clinics and still doing their surgeries. I was calling them to see how many clinics and cases they were doing that day," she says.

That evening, I called the volunteer DRC and said, 'This thing is coming to us.' He said, 'Let's wait. They are still telling us it's going to miss us. Let's wait until the 10 o'clock report comes out [from NOAA].' It was not until 11:00 P.M. when we got it. When it came out, I called him and said, 'Let's talk. We're in trouble now.' So that's when we really started looking at things."

On Saturday morning, the state alerts Cynthia's office. They need the status of every hospital—their census, supplies, staffing. Information is collected via phone, e-mail, or fax and sent to the Department of Health and Hospitals (DHH) in Baton Rouge. Area hospitals plan to set up their Incident Command Centers on Sunday, less than 24 hours before the hurricane's projected landfall. Cynthia tracks the hurricane. She believes the self-assuredness of many is because of Hurricane Georges, which had skipped the greater New Orleans area at the 11th hour.

Downtown, at City Hall on Loyola Avenue, the Emergency Operations Center (EOC) is set up. Cynthia shares office space with the city's Office of Emergency Preparedness; Entergy, Sewer and Water Board; and National Guard and Coast Guard staff. On a large whiteboard, she tracks information she receives via phone and fax from the hospitals. The plan is for every hospital to set up their Incident Command Center early Sunday morning.

On Sunday, August 28, at 4:00 A.M., New Orleans mayor C. Ray Nagin orders the first ever mandatory evacuation of New Orleans, effective at 9:00 A.M. He warns, "We're facing the storm most of us have feared." The evacuation order has exceptions that include state and federal officials, inmates of the parish prison, hospitals, hotels, and the media. At 8:00 A.M., the Superdome is opened as a shelter of last resort.

More than 1 million people evacuate from the greater New Orleans area. At noon, Cindy is notified that the last hospital has set up its Incident Command Center. As she surveys the hospitals' censuses, she becomes concerned. The number of guests in these hospitals is "astronomical," she says. "It was unbelievable how many folks were in the hospitals. In some places you had maybe 100 patients and 500 nonpatients. When I saw the numbers that were coming in, I was alarmed. These numbers included families, children, and the elderly. At that point, you begin to wonder, 'If a hospital does get hit by a big storm, who is going to be evacuated first—the patient or the family?' If you have to get them out, how are you doing that?"

At 4:00 P.M., the National Weather Service issues a special hurricane warning. The projection of possible storm impact is sobering information. In the event of a Category 4 or 5 storm, "most of the area will be uninhabitable for weeks, perhaps longer . . . At least one-half of well-constructed homes will have roof and wall failure. All gabled roofs will fail, leaving those homes severely damaged or destroyed. . . . Power outages will last for weeks . . . water shortages will make human suffering incredible by human standards" (About.com, 2005).

The status reports from the hospitals slowly come to the EOC. It is almost 7:00 P.M. when Cynthia receives the last hospital report. As Katrina tears its way through the area, communications between the EOC and hospitals become difficult as the power supply at the hospitals is taken out.

By Monday morning, August 29, the storm has passed through the area. Cynthia leaves the EOC to check on three of the downtown hospitals. There is street flooding, and she cautiously wades through water that reaches her mid-calf. She is unaware that water is pouring into the city from breaches in the levees. New Orleans is slowly drowning.

When she reaches Charity, nurses and physicians are mingling on the emergency room ramp. They report that the hospital took on a little water, but it was not too bad. At Tulane University Medical Center, she gets a similar report—minimal damage, but otherwise, everything is OK. The hospital emergency coordinator for Charity Hospital joins

Cynthia for her next stop at the VA. She finds the volunteer DRC. Most of the VA patients had been evacuated earlier. Only a few remain. Cindy and Charity's emergency coordinator resume their course and wade toward the Superdome on Poydras Street.

"I mentioned to him that the water was at my knee. I said, 'It's strange the water is a little deeper now on LaSalle Street,'" she recounts.

When they reach the Superdome, it is running on emergency generators. Inside, an estimated 25,000 people have sought shelter. Cynthia describes it as "a place with several scared people. The place was unbelievable. First we went to the Club Room, where the patients were supposed to be. There was very little light. A few emergency lights were still on. It was pretty treacherous trying to get around. Special needs patients were upstairs in the corridor area outside the Club Room because the Club Room was in total darkness. The only areas that had any light were the hallways, and walkways with very dim emergency lighting. It was heartbreaking. There were all the people in wheelchairs. Some family members were there, but not many. There were a couple of health care workers. These were all special needs, the elderly, and disabled."

There are 650 special needs patients. Many of the nurses are crying. They fear for the safety of their patients and themselves.

Cynthia says, "They are scared. Some of the patients are falling out of their wheelchairs. Others were tied into their chairs with pieces of material. Some of them had defecated in the chairs because there were only a few health workers to help them. The people that were there to take care of them were Office of Public Health nurses, who are not used to having to do hospital-type care, and they are bewildered. All of the chairs are huddled together. They weren't screaming or anything—they were just weeping."

There is no one supervising the group. Cynthia leaves to find out who is in charge. She walks down the darkened stairs and heads to the loading dock, where generator-powered floodlights shine down on a grim scene. Rows of patients lying on the floor cover the area. A National Guard unit is on-site. "I still remember this," shares Cynthia. "It looked like the scene from *Gone With the Wind*, when Scarlett is standing there looking out at all the soldiers. That is exactly what it was. It was stretcher and pallet and blanket, side by side by side."

She recognizes a physician standing in the middle of the supine patients. He sees her and asks, "What do I do?" He repeats the question. Cynthia replies, "Just try to make them as comfortable as possible." She surveys her surroundings. There are a few supply trucks by the loading dock. A large, blue tarp hangs on one side of the cavernous dock area.

At a trailer, Cynthia finds staffers conferring. The floodwaters on the back side of the Superdome are much lower than at the front, facing Poydras Street. They are trying to evacuate some of the patients.

"Nobody knew about the levees. If they did, they weren't telling anybody. I think the whole world knew the levees broke before we knew," offers Cynthia. "They are trying to see how to get the wheelchair-bound patients downstairs from the Club Room. The nonambulatory patients were downstairs.

"The escalators are very narrow, so you are not talking about a lot of space and room to move these people. But their main thrust is get help to get those people out of there. While we are in the trailer having a strategy meeting, someone keeps knocking on the door. Finally, we open the door. Eight vent-dependent patients have been brought to the Superdome without ventilators. No staffing nurses accompanied them. The group is asked what to do with these patients."

Cynthia follows them as they walk behind the hanging blue tarp. The patients range in age from the young to the elderly.

"They are lying on the ground on pallets, not stretchers. People are trying to hand-bag them. I am asked if I think they really need ventilators. I take a stethoscope and listen to breath sounds from one of the patients. I turned to them and said, 'You're in trouble. They need ventilators.'"

A physician inquires about what they are going to do. He is told, "There is nothing that can be done." They have no ventilators. Another physician insists, "We have to get ventilators." They are advised to make the patients as comfortable as they can.

Cynthia and the others return to the trailer. The situation is dire.

"Regardless if it was the ventilator patients or other ones, we have limited resources to take care of them," she states. They haven't been fed. There are no beds. Nobody knows when somebody is going to come and get them. We know that Baton Rouge says they're sending someone, but nobody really knows when they will arrive. They are still trying to figure out how they are going to get the remaining people from upstairs to downstairs. It was just a bad situation. At that point, we had been gone for a while, and I said, 'I have to return to the EOC.' We got outside. It is now 9:30, and the water is up to my thighs. I turn to him and ask, 'What's going on?'"

Cynthia struggles through the water to reach City Hall. It is dark and hard to see if there are any hazards in the water. She reaches the EOC. She learns about the breaks from a news report at 10:00 P.M. Earlier that afternoon, the mayor, from his command post at the Hyatt Hotel near the Superdome, had made a passionate plea during a live interview with WWL radio. Livid about the slow response of the federal government to the stricken city, he shouts on air, "Get off your asses and let's do something."

That evening at City Hall, Cynthia watches the news reports about the levees. She wonders why it took so long to get this critical information. She was at the Superdome when City Hall issued a 2:00 P.M. notification confirming the 17th Street levee breach that flooded 20% of the city. At 1:45 P.M., President Bush had declared emergency disaster for Louisiana and Mississippi.

"We are seeing mainly reports from the 17th Street Canal, and of course, it is from earlier in the day. We are stunned. We didn't know it. A few people who did know were with the National Guard and Coast Guard. They said yes, they got those reports. It was like they didn't believe it either," says Cynthia.

She has been in communication with the hospitals' Incident Command Centers and their corporate entities. Methodist Hospital in New Orleans East is in trouble. They have lost communications. In Mid-City, Lindy Boggs Medical Center's communications are silent as well. She knows that Chalmette Medical Center staff are aware of flooding in the region and the devastation in St. Bernard Parish. Reports start pouring into the EOC.

"For the storm, [emergency medical service] crews had all hunkered down. Some of the fire department staff was embedded at the hospitals. We are now trying to determine where they are in the field," Cynthia explains. "We start getting reports that people in the Sewerage and Water Board safe houses are not safe. One of the staffers in the EOC has a brother at the Broad Street safe house. He's getting reports the water is coming up—what are they going to do? Then they lost communication with them. I have several members of my family who work in the medical field and work in hospitals in the area. I don't know where my daughter is. I haven't been able to get a hold of her at all. I find out later that she and her boyfriend swam from the second floor of their house on Bienville Street in Mid-City. They reached the City Park off-ramp to the interstate that was at higher ground."

Because EOC is working side by side with leaders from the police and fire departments, the team can quickly verify reports as they are received. Gunfire at one hospital is determined to have come from someone in the neighborhood trying to get the attention of helicopter pilots to rescue them from their flooded home.

"Tuesday morning, I am very worried about some hospitals. I know that Lindy's got real issues, and we've lost communication with them. I also am concerned about Methodist and Chalmette. It wasn't until later

Tuesday that we got bad news about what had happened at Chalmette. We also got reports at the same time that the city government in St. Bernard had rescued them and had brought them down to the jail. So, as far as we knew, all of the patients had been cleared out of the hospital."

From City Hall, she watches the evacuation of Tulane. She is in radio contact with the VA and University Hospital. She can see the military high water trucks coming in to get the VA patients.

"[Louisiana State University's] biggest challenge was they had two campuses—Charity and University," she offers. "And their leadership people are at one hospital and they are trying to relay information between the two. But I am getting information from them. The police and the fire are telling me what's happening at Memorial, Touro, Children's. I am receiving a great amount of information, which I, in turn, am feeding to the state."

State and federal officials are focusing on the evacuation of the Convention Center and the Superdome "because as bad as the situations are at the hospitals, hospitals are still considered to be safe havens," Cynthia explains. "You've got buildings with supplies, with educated people. I think the staff at some of the hospitals got very upset. But the fact of the matter is that part of evacuation has not changed. A hospital still has to be prepared to stand in place 5–7 days because they remain a safe haven. The first tier of rescue will be for the people on top of roofs and buildings."

The state receives the information from the EOC. However, the state cannot lead and prioritize evacuation of the entire city and surrounding parishes impacted by flooding. DHH is not the leader in the search-and-rescue process.

"That is all in the hands of the military and the Wildlife and Fisheries," explains Cynthia. "So if you are at a hospital, you can keep saying, 'I want you to do this and this,' but these two groups set up their own priorities. Their viewpoint is, 'People in the hospital have got to wait.' That's just the way it is."

A frustrated Cynthia monitors the protracted evacuation process. She knows the desperate status of the hospitals waiting for their evacuation.

"At this point, I am screaming at the National Guard and Coast Guard—'They have no electricity! You can't take care of patients without electricity!' When they see me walking down the hall, they try to look for a doorway to duck into. They are probably thinking, 'There's that crazy woman,'" she says.

"But the local people, who are doing the requesting, remember they're the victims. Everyone at the local level, even the National Guard, Coast

Guard—everyone. They're in the same bowl of water that I am. So they can put out the requests, but it is still being handled out of the federal and state government levels. That's where the priorities are being set."

Universal Health Services, owner of Methodist Hospital and Chalmette Medical Center, attempts to send supplies to the two hospitals in eastern New Orleans and St. Bernard Parish. Cynthia learns that the shipment is commandeered by FEMA.

"They were commandeering everything that was coming in, because again, remember, control is now with the federal and state government. So I may say, 'I need X,' but they may think Y needs it more than I do. So they commandeer everything that comes in. They are now the ones setting priorities."

From the EOC, Cynthia watches the evacuation from Tulane University Medical Center's heliport begin on Tuesday, August 30. Airspace is now controlled by the military.

"Wednesday, the National Guard was sending out helicopters to assess the situation at Lindy and Methodist. They try to get them out first, but their mission is changed. They literally were in the air and received a change of orders. That's when I called the hospital owners and told them if they were going to get their people out anytime soon, they were going to have to do it themselves."

In the early afternoon of Thursday, September 1, Mayor Nagin issues a desperate SOS to federal officials. The city is out of resources at the Convention Center, and buses are needed.

By Saturday, September 3, hospital evacuations are complete.

Immediately after Hurricane Katrina, Cynthia joins regionwide efforts to advance emergency preparedness and communications. In January 2006, she participates in the Bring New Orleans Back Health and Social Services Committee. Significant improvements have been made, but there is need for more.

Two and a half years after Katrina, Cynthia is at City Hall for a meeting. She passes the room where EOC was stationed during the storm. Hanging on the wall is the whiteboard where she marked her updates through September 3, 2005.

"I happened to walk in that room for the first time since the storm, and my board was still there with my handwriting on it. It was shocking. I was totally taken aback," she shares. "There was the board. On it was my last entry of hospitals that had evacuated. It was a shock seeing that over 2 years later."

8   Going Forward

There have been numerous lessons learned from the events that occurred with Hurricane Katrina and the subsequent failure of the levee system. This chapter provides a glimpse of accomplishments that have occurred over the past 4 years by way of improving the many facets of emergency preparedness. These include the recent legislation enacted by the state of Louisiana, a noteworthy policy paper developed by the American Nurses Association (ANA), and standards and policies created by regulatory and accreditation agencies that will ensure that all health care organizations and professionals, and city and state stakeholders, are in a state of readiness for any man-made or natural disaster.

Since 9/11, there have been continued efforts to improve emergency preparedness across the nation. Among these improvements are policy development, improvement of emergency management standards, identification of competencies needed for health care providers, and federal and state legislation that establishes improvement for health care workers facing inevitable disasters.

AMERICAN NURSES ASSOCIATION POLICY PAPER

Due to the aftermath of Hurricane Katrina and the conditions nurses faced providing care during such an emergency, the ANA identified the dilemma of how health care professionals, and in particular, nurses, are faced with concerns related to the standard of care. As a result, in June 2007, the ANA convened a national policy conference called "Nursing Care in Life, Death, and Disaster" to engage health care professionals across the country on policy issues related to disaster and emergency management. Generated by the feedback of conference participants, recommendations from an expert panel, and a review of the state and national guidelines for standards of care (ANA Code of Ethics for Nurses, ANA Standards of Practice and Standards of Professional Performance, National Incident Management System [NIMS]), a policy document titled, *Adapting Standards of Care Under Extreme Conditions: Guidance for Professionals During Disasters, Pandemics, and Other Extreme Emergencies* was developed (ANA, 2008).

This policy document serves as a guide for health care providers who are faced with caring for patients under extreme circumstances due to a change in available resources (loss of water and/or electricity), a change in practice setting (alternate unit or facility), or a change in the type and number of patients requiring care. Even with these changes, health care professionals must be prepared to adapt to these changes and provide the best possible care to patients. This does not mean that professional competencies and standards of care and practice change in an emergency event. Every nurse has a professional obligation to be personally and legally accountable for actions taken in the course of professional nursing practice.

The Center for Public Health Preparedness (2003) at Columbia University School of Nursing and the Nursing Education Education Preparedness Coalition (2003) have developed competencies for emergency preparedness and response for nurses. These documents assert that these competencies apply to all professional nurse roles in all practice areas, but the knowledge and ability to perform certain duties and tasks during a disaster are contingent on the functional role of each individual nurse as well as on educational preparation and type of practice setting. The ANA policy document asserts that during the period of providing care under extreme circumstances, certain priorities need to be addressed. These priorities include maintaining patient and worker safety, maintaining essential bodily functions (airway, breathing, circulation, and blood loss), and maintaining infection control. Care issues that may be left for a later time include routine care (i.e. turning, ambulation), administration of oral medications, extensive documentation of care, maintenance of complete privacy and confidentiality, and elective procedures.

The ANA policy paper provides recommendations for the emergency event by providing an outline of certain activities that individual registered nurses or other health care professionals, health care facilities or other practice sites, and emergency response planners should complete in each of the phases of pre-event, event, and postevent. Some of the activities that individual registered nurses or other health care professionals should accomplish include becoming knowledgeable about the NIMS and National Response Plan, providing the best care to the patients, and participation in postevent evaluation (ANA, 2008). Health care facilities and practice sites should develop a plan to use volunteers, provide just-in-time training for staff, and participate in postevent evaluation (ANA, 2008). The focus on emergency response planners ensures that health care facilities are involved in emergency planning related to legal declarations of emergencies and participate in postevent evaluation (ANA, 2008).

The ANA policy paper is a fundamental document that all health care professionals, particularly nurses, should be aware of and use as a resource, especially when preparing for a disaster. The paper is simply a guideline, and the first attempt of nursing's professional organization to provide guidelines that health care professionals and organizations may use to prepare in a disaster. The ANA has developed valuable information on bioterrorism and disaster response that can be located on the ANA's Web site. Topics include how to care for patients, action alerts, and the national nurse's response team.

Additional education available for emergency and disaster training includes the National Disaster Life Support (NDLS) education program, sponsored by the American Medical Association (AMA; n.d.), and the NIMS educational programs. The AMA developed a certification program, the National Disaster Life Support Program, that focuses on the all-hazards approach to emergency preparedness and response. The program contains a Basic Disaster Life Support course and an Advanced Disaster Life Support course. NIMS provides a model for incident management (Federal Emergency Management Agency, 2008). NIMS courses are available online and consist of multiple courses, ranging from basic to advanced. The Federal Emergency Management Agency

(FEMA) has a 5-year NIMS Training Plan that incorporates multiple aspects of compliance training, addressing such objectives as communications and information management and Incident Command Systems. It is the responsibility of every health care organization and health care professional to prepare prior to a disaster to minimize damage, and to use minimum resources that may result in proficiency and effectiveness. It should be noted that health care professionals realize that providing care under extreme conditions may warrant using the limited resources that they have to make decisions based on saving those whose recovery is more likely.

THE JOINT COMMISSION

The Joint Commission is an independent nonprofit organization that was founded in 1951 by the American College of Physicians, the American Hospital Association, the AMA, and the Canadian Medical Association, in collaboration with the American College of Surgeons (Joint Commission, 2009), to provide voluntary accreditation of health care organizations. The American College of Surgeons created the minimum standards for hospitals in 1917. In 1952, the American College of Surgeons transitioned the Hospital Standardization Program to the Joint Commission Accreditation of Hospitals (JCAH), which started offering the accreditation program to hospitals in 1953 (Joint Commission, 2009). The Joint Commission has a long history, since its inception, of establishing performance standards to measure quality, performance improvement, and outcomes through accreditation and certification of health care organizations. The Joint Commission also has a mission of inclusiveness and the education of health care personnel with a transparency that focuses on quality improvement.

In 2007, due to major disasters across the country, such as hurricanes, floods, and tornados, the Joint Commission realized that the emergency management standards and guidelines required revision for hospitals, critical access hospitals, and long-term care programs. The Joint Commission identified six crucial areas that, if addressed, would create an all-hazards approach to emergency preparedness and response. These critical areas included communication, safety and security, staff roles and responsibilities, utilities, clinical and support activities, and resources and assets. If the health care facilities prepare by using these critical areas of emergency management for outcomes, better outcomes may be achieved. It is each health care organization's responsibility to adhere to these standards (Joint Commission, 2008).

The Joint Commission, along with the Joint Commission Resources, have developed and published several useful documents addressing emergency management. During Hurricane Katrina in 2005, many facilities became overwhelmed with the number of patients (i.e., hundreds and thousands) seeking care or shelter. These facilities did not have the capacity, due to physical constraints (i.e., size of facility, damages), to take in additional patients. In an effort to address this daunting issue, in its publication titled, *Surge Hospitals: Providing Safe Care in Emergencies*, the Joint Commission (2005b) describes the types of surge hospitals that can be expanded to care for a large influx of patients, including closed hospitals and nursing units and departments, portable and mobile facilities, and nonmedical buildings, which can be converted to function as medical facilities.

The second document, *Standing Together—An Emergency Planning Guide for America's Communities*, was developed because of the constraints on, and lack of resources of, many small rural and suburban communities when confronted with the task of supporting themselves for days following a disaster (Joint Commission, 2005a). It is a comprehensive and in-depth document that describes the challenges that rural communities may have to address, explains how to develop community-wide preparedness plans that are inclusive of both private and public partnerships, and provides tools and Web sites to use as resources.

The third document, developed from a round table and national symposium and titled *Health Care at the Crossroads: Strategies for Creating and Sustaining Community-wide Emergency Preparedness Systems* (Joint Commission, 2003), is the result of the Joint Commission's work on their Public Policy Initiative to address emergency preparedness stemming from the terrorist attacks of 9/11. This document addresses the responsibilities of both federal and state governments in emergency preparedness and also provides specific recommendations for issues identified by the round table and symposium participants. Under the general topics that are detailed, recommendations include enlisting the community in preparing the local response, determining what is needed for the community to maintain resources to care for patients, protecting the staff and serving the public, and creating the accountability of leaders.

The Joint Commission has a wealth of information available to health care professionals and organizations, community members, and the public in preparing for any man-made or natural disaster.

LEGISLATION

Since 2005, state and federal legislation regarding emergency and disaster management has been developed. Several of the laws that have been enacted on a national level include the National Disaster Relief Act of 2008, part of the Emergency Economic Stabilization Act of 2008; the Pets Evacuation and Transportation Standards Act of 2006; and the Disaster Recovery Personal Protection Act of 2006. The National Disaster Relief Act of 2008 was signed into law on October 3, 2008. This legislation provides tax relief for disaster victims after December 31, 2007, and before January 1, 2010.

The Pets Evacuation and Transportation Standards Act was passed at both federal and state levels. Congress passed this legislation on October 6, 2006; the legislation requires FEMA to ensure that at both local and state levels, pets are included in the evacuation plans. The Disaster Recovery Personal Protection Act was passed into law at the federal level. This law prohibits all levels of the government, federal, state, and local, from confiscating lawfully owned firearms during a declared emergency status.

The state of Louisiana, including the greater New Orleans area, has developed a comprehensive emergency preparedness plan, along with many resources now available to health care providers and citizens. The Office of Louisiana Homeland Security and Emergency Preparedness, under the Governor's Office, along with both the Louisiana Senate and House of Representatives, was created to provide leadership and assistance for improving emergency preparedness planning and readiness, thereby ensuring that citizens are safe and secure throughout the state.

Due to the catastrophic events that occurred with Hurricane Katrina and the failure of the levee system, the state of Louisiana took the initiative of reforming disaster medicine laws. HB 1379-2008 Regular Session was signed by the governor as Act 758, with an effective date of August 15, 2008, and titled the Health/Emergency Medical Service (Louisiana State Legislature, 2008). It addresses the issue that medical personnel may be involved in complex medical issues during an emergency. It acknowledges that in a disaster situation, medical personnel are under intense pressure, with limited resources, and that an independent emergency/disaster medicine review panel is to review the conduct of medical personnel regarding clinical judgment during a disaster and provide an independent and objective advisory opinion. Act 758 states,

To enact R.S. 29:735.3 and R.S. 40:1299.39.3, relative to health-care services rendered during an emergency; to provide for legislative findings and intent; to provide for a review of health-care services rendered during a state of emergency prior to criminal prosecution; to provide for an Emergency/ Disaster Medicine Review Panel; to provide for membership of the review panel; to provide for a procedure for the review of health care services rendered during the state of emergency; to provide for definitions; to provide with respect to confidentiality; and to provide for related matters. (Louisiana State Legislature, 2008, p. 1)

In addition, Act 758 asserts that the information provided by the review panel will be used by the prosecuting authority to determine if good-faith judgment of the health care provider was used in the care provided and to prevent future untoward occurrences from impacting future patients in an emergency event.

Presented earlier were a few of the initiatives enacted since Hurricane Katrina to strengthen and improve overall preparedness and response to such a disaster. There are several more not covered in this book. One last issue to address is the ongoing economic recovery of the Gulf Coast after Hurricane Katrina. The Department of Commerce has published six reports regarding economic recovery post-Katrina. *The Gulf Coast: Economic Recovery Two Years After the Hurricanes* (Economics and Statistics Administration, 2007) provides insight regarding the economic recovery that has occurred since the hurricanes decimated the infrastructure of New Orleans and its people. Overall, the economic recovery is improving in the state of Louisiana, but economic conditions in New Orleans are lagging behind. Of particular interest to health care professionals is the public assistance funding offered by FEMA, consisting of $442 million of the $503 million needed to rebuild the infrastructure of health care in Louisiana. According to the report, out of 550 storm-damaged health care structures, about 500 have resumed services. Other economic indicators, specifically for New Orleans, note that the New Orleans metropolitan service area has not recovered to its prehurricane population, occupied housing remains significantly lower than its pre-Katrina levels, industry output increased in construction and durable goods manufacturing, the labor force is 20% below pre-Katrina levels, employment levels among the labor force are 80% of pre-Katrina levels, and tourism is showing a steady increase. As a whole, the economic indicators are moving in a slow positive direction for the city of New Orleans.

LESSONS LEARNED

Since Hurricane Katrina, numerous lessons have been learned and improvements made in emergency and disaster preparedness and readiness. Such identified improvements include the following:

- *Improvements in organizations' emergency preparedness plans.* Because of the need for improvements in health care organizational preparedness plans, in 2008, the Joint Commission identified six critical areas (communication, safety and security, staff roles and responsibilities, utilities, clinical and support activities, and resources and assets) on which to focus in managing any emergency or disaster situation. These critical areas create an all-hazards approach to emergency and disaster management. Several examples of improvements in these six critical areas include the following:
  - Because of the number of patients and other individuals (visitors, family members, volunteers) inside facilities during the Hurricane Katrina disaster, there was an increased need to protect the facility and people who were housed there. As a result, health care organizations developed facility lockdown procedures, implemented curfews, and identified a need for stronger internal security by hiring additional security officers from outside resources.
  - Hospitals have purchased special evacuation devices and equipment because of the need to transport and evacuate patients, particularly nonambulatory individuals, during a disaster. Examples of evacuation devices and equipment purchased include evacuation sleds and chairs, transport chairs for stairwell use, and motorized boats.
  - Structural plant modifications have been made in hospitals because of the loss of generator power and significant damage to the overall facility structure caused by flooding. Such structural plant modifications include moving generators above the ground floor to eliminate the risk of flooding them; purchasing portable generators to connect to the facility's main power source when a disaster occurs; relocating the transfer switches and power distribution control subpanels that feed the power to the facility above the ground floor; hardening the facility,

which includes building flood walls around certain areas of the facility and building dykes around the power plant; drilling a water well next to the facility to ensure a water supply; and repairing or building new heliports to support air evacuation of victims.

■ Since evacuation of patients is initially the responsibility of the state and local governments, and due to the lack of an adequate plan for evacuating individuals needing assistance, a local, regional, and state approach to patient evacuation for both in-state and out-of-state movement of patients was instituted. Each of the nine regions in Louisiana has a designated regional coordinator who works in collaboration with the facilities in identifying resources to assist with evacuation and transfers. The state has identified a timeline for hospital evacuations, where H-hour (landfall of the hurricane) is the decisive factor.

■ Due to the lack of coordination and documentation of the transfer and evacuation of patients, a statewide patient tracking and locater system was implemented. A Web site was created by the Louisiana Hospital Association to collect data on the identification of patients who are moved during a disaster. Hospitals provide the association with a list of patients who are transferred and evacuated.

■ Due to the decimation of the communication infrastructure post–Hurricane Katrina, the state of Louisiana implemented the EMSystem Resource Tracking Program and an emergency alert system. The EMSystem Resource Tracking Program is a tool that can be used to prepare for emergencies and disasters through its alert and notification mechanism, and the system can provide a current census of patients by patient type (medical/surgical, pediatric, etc.) in both the emergency department and hospital-wide. The emergency alert system, NOLAReady, is a text-messaging system that individuals can sign up with and thereby receive text messages from city officials regarding impending emergency situations such as dangerous weather, amber alerts, or evacuation and shelter in place information.

■ *Disaster competencies for health care personnel.* Since nurses and other health care providers provide a crucial role in emergency and disaster management, it is essential that they acquire the needed skills and abilities to respond successfully in such situations.

Documents such as the *ICN Framework of Disaster Nursing Competencies* (World Health Organization & International Council of Nurses, 2009) or the *Emergency Preparedness and Response Competencies for Hospital Workers* (Center for Public Health Preparedness, 2003) provide a framework for education and training of health care professionals for disaster situations.

■ *Disaster education.* It is imperative that health care professionals be prepared prior to a disaster. Educational programs, both formally, in schools of nursing and other academic settings, and informally, including online educational courses addressing emergency and disaster training (e.g., NIMS National Disaster Life Support Program) for students, health care professionals, and individuals in the public, private, and governmental sectors, are available. The FEMA Emergency Management Higher Education Program provides information about disaster and emergency management to universities and colleges.

■ *Laws and regulations affecting emergency and disaster management.* Nurses and other health care professionals must be knowledgeable about laws and regulations regarding the provision of care for individuals during an emergency and disaster. Since 2005, federal and state legislation has been enacted to address emergency and disaster management. Such legislation includes several laws:

  ■ The Health/Emergency Medical Service, Act 758 (Louisiana State Legislature, 2008), acknowledges that medical personnel are under extreme pressure, with limited resources, during a disaster and that an independent emergency/disaster medicine review panel will be established to review the conduct of medical personnel regarding clinical judgment during a disaster, providing an independent and objective advisory opinion.

  ■ The Uniform Emergency Volunteer Health Practitioners Act, Act 397 (Louisiana State Legislature, 2009), allows for licensed health care professionals to volunteer across state lines when an emergency/disaster has been declared by the governor. Specific requirements that the licensed health care professional must adhere to are outlined in Act 397, such as signing up with an interstate compact in advance of the declared emergency/disaster to become eligible as a volunteer. In addition, the law does provide for a limit of liability for volunteers.

- The Disaster Recovery Personal Protection Act protects against the confiscation of lawfully owned firearms during a declared emergency situation.
- The National Disaster Relief Act addresses tax relief measures for disaster victims.
- The Pets Evacuation and Transportation Standards Act address the evacuation of pets in a disaster.

- *Louisiana Hospital Emergency Preparedness and Response Plan (2007).* Due to the devastation that hurricanes Katrina and Rita brought to Louisiana, the state developed an infrastructure to successfully respond to disasters by improving the hospital emergency preparedness and response plan. Examples of improvements made to the plan include the following:

  - A regional structure was created to have a multitiered response in the way local health care organizations are prepared to function in a disaster. Each hospital is placed in one of the nine regions.
  - Criteria were developed for hospitals based on services that can be provided during a disaster: designated regional hospitals (larger acute hospitals, emergency room services, and surge facilities), Tier 1 hospitals (have emergency services 24/7), and Tier 2 hospitals (no emergency room services and focus on one modality).
  - The establishment of ongoing drills, both announced and unannounced, was undertaken to ensure that the health care organizations are in a state of readiness.

- Resources
  - The Joint Commission has numerous resources available that addresses emergency and disaster management. Among these are the publications *Surge Hospitals: Providing Safe Care in Emergencies* (Joint Commission, 2005b), *Standing Together— An Emergency Planning Guide for America's Communities* (Joint Commission, 2005a), and *Emergency Preparedness: Healthcare at the Crossroads: Strategies for Creating and Sustaining Community-wide Emergency Preparedness Systems* (Joint Commission, 2003). These documents provide valuable information for health care organizations and communities preparing for any type of emergency or disaster.

- The ANA's (2008) policy document titled *Adapting Standards of Care Under Extreme Conditions: Guidance for Professionals During Disasters, Pandemics, and Other Extreme Emergencies* addresses the concerns raised by many nurses after Hurricane Katrina regarding the ethical and practice issues that arise when nurses are faced with caring for people in devastating situations.

- Several congressional and governmental reports identify improvements needed from the lessons learned following Hurricane Katrina. One such report, *The Federal Response to Hurricane Katrina: Lessons Learned* (White House, 2006), highlights 125 recommendations for improvement from the lessons learned during this disaster. These relate to improving national preparedness by understanding and becoming knowledgeable on the National Response Plan, developing a National Emergency Communications Strategy, creating a logistics system that coordinates with the public and private sectors, assisting in large-scale evacuations when the state and local governments are not able to manage such a task, and guaranteeing that a federal law enforcement response is implemented. Several other reports emphasize the same critical flaws that occurred during this disaster.

There are many more lessons learned, but not included here, from the events that occurred during one of the largest disasters in U.S. history: Hurricane Katrina. It is hoped that they will provide useful information to assist in the continued training and education of health care professionals so that we can provide for the needs of people in times of disaster.

Epilogue

The scope of Hurricane Katrina's devastation was unprecedented. In the greater New Orleans area, every hospital was impacted to some degree. Local, state, and federal government officials faced a daunting job in rescuing thousands of people. Hurricane Katrina overwhelmed residents and government officials at the local, state, and federal levels alike. Emergency responders at all levels of government were inundated with rescue requests from throughout the area.

In the days immediately following Hurricane Katrina, the flooded hospitals in the greater New Orleans area faced a major task—total evacuation. Power lines and phones were out. Cell towers were down, and few cell phones had reception. Every day they stayed in place, the hospitals' staffs faced further depletion of food and water supplies. Fuel for emergency generators would eventually run out.

The staff knew that there were other facilities in the same predicament. That knowledge was consoling, and also a sobering reality. How do you evacuate several hospitals that are now islands? When the water surrounding your medical campus is several feet deep, evacuation is by boat or air. There are no other options.

In a disaster, we are almost always our own first responders because there is no guarantee that official help will arrive quickly enough. Communications are a lifeline. Response to the situation is guided by the communications received. The hurricane fueled misinformation at all levels. Chasing information and separating fact from rumor became a critical, yet frustrating, exercise.

Inside these hospitals, the oppressive August heat was unforgiving. Temperatures soared above 100°. Nurses, physicians, employees, and volunteers worked to exhaustion helping with patient evacuation, and then their own evacuation. Many knew that their homes had been destroyed by the flooding, yet they put aside thoughts about personal loss and focused on the job and its urgency—getting everyone out.

In addition to caring for their patients, nurses also treated people who sought refuge at their hospitals. While nurses have always faced the possibility and eventuality of working under altered conditions during both natural and man-made disasters, nurses who worked through the altered conditions forced on them by Katrina were irrevocably affected. Many nurses did not return to bedside nursing. Others never returned to the region.

Katrina inflicted numerous levels of loss and many degrees of human suffering. It was also a catalyst for improvement. The private sector and government are focused on improved communications and cooperation. Investments have been made in technology to ensure that communications are maintained in a disaster. Legislation has been passed—the National Disaster Relief Act of 2008, the Pets Evacuation and Transportation Standards Act of 2006, and the Disaster Recovery Personal Protection Act of 2006.

The emergency response to Hurricane Katrina will be dissected and analyzed for years to come. Those who say Katrina is history and that it is time to move on discount the conditions under which these flooded hospitals operated. The purpose of this book has been to try to provide a more complete picture of the nurses' Katrina experience so that we can move forward.

References

About.com. (2005, August 28). *NOAA urgent weather message from NWS New Orleans.* Retrieved September 4, 2009, from http://stormtrack.blogspot.com/2005/08/urgent-weather-message-from-nws-new.html

American Medical Association. (n.d.). *The National Disaster Life Support Program.* Retrieved January 10, 2009, from http://www.ama-assn.org/ama/pub/physician-resources/public-health/center-public-health-preparedness-disaster-response/national-disaster-life-support.shtml

American Nurses Association. (2008). *Adapting standards of care under extreme conditions: Guidance for professionals during disasters, pandemics, and other extreme emergencies.* Silver Spring, MD: Author.

American Society of Civil Engineers. (2007). *The New Orleans Hurricane Protection System: What went wrong and why.* Retrieved June 5, 2009, from http://www.asce.org/static/hurricane/whitehouse.cfm

Bazile, K. (2007, February 13). *Chalmette Hospital reduced to rubble.* Retrieved June 11, 2009, from http://www.nola.com/news/t-p/metro/index.ssf?/base/news-19/1171351267298340.xml&coll=1

Carter, N., & Stern, C. (2006, August 4). *Mississippi River Gulf Outlet (MRGO): Issues for Congress* (Congressional Research Service Report No. RL 33597). Retrieved June 10, 2009, from http://ncseonline.org/NLE/crs/abstract.cfm?NLEid=1728

Center for Public Health Preparedness. (2003). *Emergency preparedness and response competencies for hospital workers.* Retrieved June 11, 2009, from Columbia University Web site: http://www.ncdp.mailman.columbia.edu/files/hospcomps.pdf

Congressional Hazards Caucus. (2008, June 19). *Levee protection: Working with the geology and environment to build resiliency.* Retrieved June 11, 2009, from http://www.hazardscaucus.org/briefings/levees_briefing0608.html

Dawes, D., & Nolan, C. (2004). *Religious pioneers: Building the faith in the Archdiocese of New Orleans.* New Orleans, LA: Roman Catholic Church of the Archdiocese of New Orleans.

DeGregorio, J. (2007, December 24). Pact seals the demise of Mid-city hospital. *Times Picayune. http://www.nola.com/news/index.ssf/2007/12/pact_seals_demise_of_midcity_h.html*

Disaster Recovery Personal Protection Act of 2006, H.R. 5013, 109th Cong. (2006).

Economics and Statistics Administration. (2007, December). *The Gulf Coast: Economic recovery two years after the hurricanes.* Retrieved June 8, 2009, from http://www.eda.gov/PDF/GulfCoast2yr20808.pdf

Emergency Economic Stabilization Act of 2008, H.R. 1424, 110th Cong. (2007).

Environmental News Service. (2006, April 6). *California advances funds to Army Corps for critical levee repair.* Retrieved June 10, 2009, from http://www.ens-newswire.com/ens/apr2006/2006-04-06-04.asp

Federal Emergency Management Agency. (2008). *NIMS resource center.* Retrieved May 1, 2009, from http://www.fema.gov/emergency/nims/

Finch, S. (2009, April 20). Entries from latest metro New Orleans news tagged with "flooding." *Times-Picayune,* p. B1.

Greene, G. (1976). *The history of Southern Baptist Hospital* (Rev. ed.). New Orleans, LA: Southern Baptist Hospital.

Grissett, S. (2009, May 3). Army Corps of Engineers' pump plans for three New Orleans outfall canals surge ahead. *Times-Picayune,* p. A5.

H. Rep. No. 109-377 (2006).

Hanggi-Myers, L. (1996). The origins and history of the first public health/community health nurses in Louisiana 1835–1927 (Doctoral dissertation, Louisiana State University Health Sciences Center School of Nursing, 1996). *Dissertation Abstracts International, 22,* 185–193.

Homeland Security and Governmental Affairs Senate Committee. (2005a, November 2). *Senate Homeland Security Committee holds Hurricane Katrina hearing to examine levees in New Orleans.* Retrieved June 11, 2009, from http://hsgac.senate.gov/public/index.cfm?FuseAction=PressReleases.Detail&Affiliation=R&PressRelease_id=10b8e67d-fe83-4d81-ac29-aba3d1e6d425&Month=11&Year=2005

Homeland Security and Governmental Affairs Senate Committee. (2005b, December 15). *Hurricane Katrina: Who's in charge of the New Orleans levees?* Retrieved June 11, 2009, from http://hsgac.senate.gov/public/_files/121505SMCOpen.pdf

Infrastructure Security Partnership. (2002–2009). *U.S. Army Corps of Engineers Interagency Performance Evaluation Task Force (IPET) releases final DRA.* Retrieved June 11, 2009, from http://tisp.org/index.cfm?cdid=10754&pid=10260

Joint Commission. (2003, March). *Health care at the crossroads: Strategies for creating and sustaining community-wide emergency preparedness systems.* Retrieved June 6, 2009, from http://www.jointcommission.org/PublicPolicy/Emergency_Preparedness.htm

Joint Commission. (2005a, November). *Standing together—An emergency planning guide for America's communities.* Retrieved June 6, 2009, from http://www.jointcommission.org/PublicPolicy/ep_guide.htm

Joint Commission. (2005b, December). *Surge hospitals: Providing safe care in emergencies.* Retrieved June 6, 2009, from http://www.jointcommission.org/PublicPolicy/surge_hospitals.htm

Joint Commission. (2008). *2008 hospital accreditation standards.* Oak Terrace, IL: Author.

Joint Commission. (2009). *A journey through the history of Joint Commission.* Retrieved June 6, 2009, from http://www.jointcommission.org/AboutUs/joint_commission_history.htm

Kennedy, D. (2005, September 2). *NPR's unlikely pit bull.* Retrieved March 10, 2009, from http://medianation.blogspot.com/2005/09/nprs-unlikely-pit-bull.html

Louisiana Hospital Association. (2007). *HHS emergency preparedness.* Retrieved May 10, 2009, from http://www.lhaonline.org/displaycommon.cfm?an=1&subarticlenbr=138

Louisiana State Legislature. (2008). *Act 758.* Retrieved June 3, 2009, from http://www.legis.state.la.us/billdata/byinst.asp?sessionid=08rs&billtype=HB&billno=1379

Louisiana State Legislature. (2009). *Act 397*. Retrieved July 13, 2009, from http://www.legis.state.la.us/billdata/streamdocument.asp?did=668826

Methodist Health System Foundation Inc. (2008). *MHSF annual report: July 1, 2007–June 30, 2008*. Retrieved September 2, 2009, from http://www.mhsfi.org/about_us/annual_report/

National Disaster Relief Act of 2008 (2008). http://thomas.loc.gov/cgi-bin/query/F?c110:1:./temp/~c110C1uvXQ:e499915

National Hurricane Center. (2005a). *Hurricane Katrina advisory number 26*. Retrieved May 20, 2009, from http://www.nhc.noaa.gov/archive/2005/pub/al122005.public_026.shtml

National Hurricane Center. (2005b, August 29). *Hurricane Katrina advisory number 27A*. Retrieved June 6, 2009, from http://www.nhc.noaa.gov/archive/2005/pub/al122005.public_a.026.shtml

Nursing Emergency Preparedness Education Coalition. (2003). *Educational competencies for registered nurses responding to mass casualty incidents*. Retrieved July 8, 2009, from http://www.nursing.vanderbilt.edu/incmce/competencies.html

Pets Evacuation and Transportation Standards Act of 2006, H.R. 3858, 109th Cong. (2006).

S. Rep. No. 109-322 (2006).

Salavaggio, J. (1992). *New Orleans' Charity Hospital: A story of physicians, politics and poverty*. Baton Rouge: Louisiana State University Press.

Schleifstein, M. (2009). U.S. Sen. Mary Landrieu: U.S. should adopt Netherlands-like policies for flood control. *Times-Picayune*, A3. Retrieved September 14, 2009, from http://www.nola.com/news/index.ssf/2009/06/us_sen_mary_landrieu_us_should.html

Seed, R., Bea, R., Abdelmalak, R., Athanasopoulos, A., Boutwell, G., Bray, J., et al. (2006). *Investigation of the performance of the New Orleans flood protection systems*. Retrieved June 10, 2009, from http://www.ce.berkeley.edu/projects/neworleans/report/VOL_1.pdf

Sisters of Mercy of the Americas. (2006a). *Catherine McAuley*. Retrieved February 21, 2009, from http://www.sistersofmercy.org/index.php?option=com_content&task=view&id=109&Ite

Sisters of Mercy of the Americas. (2006b). *Mercy comes to America*. Retrieved February 21, 2009, from http://www.sistersofmercy.org/index.php?option=com_content&task=view&id=108&Itemid=163

Southern Baptist Convention Annual (1921). In G. Greene (1976), The history of Southern Baptist Hospital (Rev. ed.). pp 35-36. New Orleans, LA: Southern Baptist Hospital.

St. Bernard Parish. (1999, June 20). *Future development*. Retrieved June 10, 2009, from http://www.enlou.com/econ/stbernard_econ.htm

University Hospital. (1996–2007). *History*. Retrieved June 1, 2009, from http://www.mclno.org/MCLNO//Menu/Hospital/History/UniversityHistory.aspx

U.S. Army Corps of Engineers Team New Orleans. (n.d.). *Mississippi River Gulf Outlet (MRGO) closure*. Retrieved June 10, 2009, from http://www.mvn.usace.army.mil/pd/projectsList/home.asp?projectID=164

U.S. Government Accountability Office. (2005, September 28). *Army Corps of Engineers: Lake Pontchartrain and Vicinity Hurricane Protection Project*. Retrieved June 11, 2009, from http://www.gao.gov/products/GAO-05-1050T

U.S. House of Representatives. (2006). *Select bipartisan committee to investigate the preparation for and response to Hurricane Katrina.* Retrieved June 7, 2009, from http://katrina.house.gov/full_katrina_report.htm

White House. (2006, February). *The federal response to Hurricane Katrina: Lessons learned.* Retrieved June 5, 2009, from http://georgewbush-whitehouse.archives.gov/reports/katrina-lessons-learned/

Wooley, D., & Shabman, L. (2007). *Decision-making chronology for Lake Pontchartrain and Vicinity Hurricane Protection Project.* Retrieved June 11, 2009, from http://graphics8.nytimes.com/packages/pdf/national/20070711_HPDC.pdf

World Health Organization & International Council of Nurses. (2009). *ICN framework of disaster nursing competencies.* Geneva, Switzerland: World Health Organization Western Pacific Region.

Bibliography

BOOKS

Barry, J. (1997). *Rising tide: The great Mississippi flood of 1927 and how it changed America.* New York: Touchstone.

Bergal, J., Hiles, S., Koughan, F., McQuaid, J., Morris, J., Reckdahl, K., et al. (2007). *City adrift: New Orleans before and after Katrina.* Baton Rouge: Louisiana State University Press.

Buuck, M. (2008). *The St. Bernard Fire Department in Hurricane Katrina.* Gretna, LA: Pelican.

Dallas Morning News. (2005). *Eyes of the storm: Hurricanes Katrina and Rita: The photographic story.* Lanham, MD: Taylor Trade.

Gannett Inc. (2005). *Katrina: Devastation. Survival. Restoration. (A unique look through the eyes of 40 photojournalists).* McLean, VA: Gannett.

Garvey, J., & Widmer, M. (1982). *Beautiful crescent: A history of New Orleans.* New Orleans, LA: Garmer Press.

Honoré, R. (2009). *Survival: How a culture of preparedness can save you and your family from disasters.* New York: Atria.

Horne, J. (2006). *Breach of faith: Hurricane Katrina and the near death of a great American city.* New York: Random House.

Larsen, E. (2000). *Isaac's storm: A man, a time, and the deadliest hurricane in history.* New York: Vintage Books.

Moyé, L. (2006). *Face to face with Katrina survivors: A first responder's tribute.* Greensboro, NC: Open Hand.

Ory, C., & Thompson, B. (2006). *Disconnected: A true Hurricane Katrina story.* Mustang, OK: Tate.

Tidwell, M. (2006). *The ravaging tide: Strange weather, future Katrina and the coming death of America's coastal cities.* New York: Free Press.

Van Heerden, I., & Bryan, M. (2006). *The storm: What went wrong and why during Hurricane Katrina. The inside story from one Louisiana scientist.* New York: Penguin Group.

Yoes, P. (2006). *Chest deep and rising: The Hurricane Katrina nightmare.* New York: Ithaca.

PAPERS

Agency for Healthcare Research and Quality. (2007). *Bioterrorism and other public health emergencies: Tools for planning and preparedness.* Retrieved June 11, 2009, from http://www.ahrq.gov/prep/

Agency for Healthcare Research and Quality. (2007). *Emergency preparedness atlas: U.S. nursing home and hospital facilities* (AHRQ Publication No. 07-0029-2). Retrieved June 11, 2009, from http://www.ahrq.gov/prep/nursinghomes/atlas.htm

Federal Emergency Management Agency. (1996). *All hazards planning guide.* Retrieved June 9, 2009, from http://www.fema.gov/pdf/plan/0-prelim.pdf

Federal Emergency Management Agency. (2004). *Are you ready? An in depth guide to citizen preparedness.* Retrieved June 9, 2009, from http://www.fema.gov/areyouready/

Gray, B., & Hebert, K. (2006). *After Katrina: Hospitals in Hurricane Katrina.* Washington, D.C.: The Urban Institute.

Johnson, D. (2006). *Service assessment: Hurricane Katrina August 23–31, 2005.* Silver Spring, MD: National Oceanic and Atmospheric Administration.

U.S. Department of Health and Human Services. (2007). *Public health emergency response: A guide for leaders and responders.* Retrieved June 9, 2009, from http://www.hhs.gov/disasters/press/newsroom/leadersguide/index.html

U.S. Department of Veterans Affairs. (2008, February 5). *Emergency management principles and practices for health care systems.* Retrieved June 8, 2009, from http://www1.va.gov/emshg/page.cfm?pg=122

PERIODICALS

National Geographic. (2005, December). Katrina: Why it became a man-made disaster, where it could happen next [Special issue]. *National Geographic.*

WEB SITES

American Nurses Association, http://nursingworld.org/

American Red Cross, http://www.redcross.org/

Center for the Study of Public Health Impacts of Hurricanes, http://www.publichealth.hurricane.lsu.edu

Coalition to Restore Coastal Louisiana, from http://www.crcl.org/

Emergency Management Agency, http://www.fema.gov/

Emergency Nurses Association, http://www.ena.org/practice/EmergencyPrepared/Pages/Default.aspx

Levees.org, http://www.levees.org/

Louisiana Homeland Security and Emergency Preparedness, http://www.ohsep.louisiana.gov/

National Academy of Engineering, http://www.nae.edu/

National Hurricane Center, http://www.nhc.noaa.gov/

Times Picayune, Washing Away Series, http://www.nola.com/hurricane/??washingaway/

Index

.